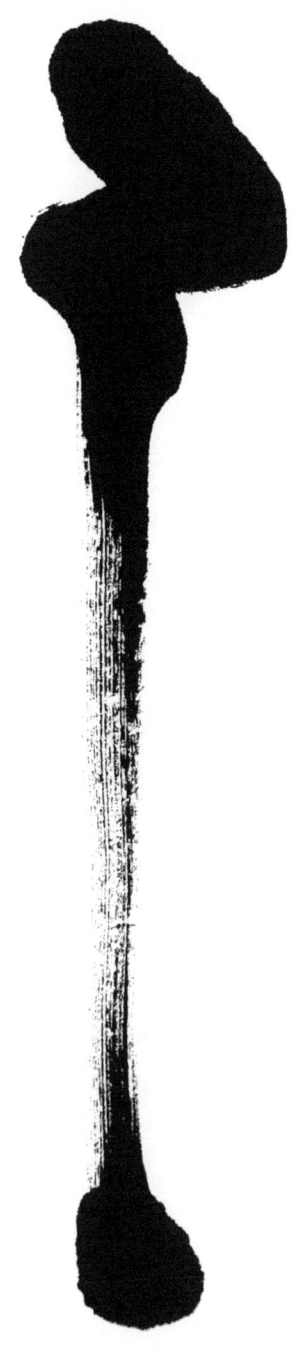

FACING SUFFERING

Gordon M. Greene

Water Margin Press, Spring Green, Wisconsin
2nd Edition, 2020
ISBN: 978-1-7341373-1-6

Table of Contents

Foreword _____ vii

Introduction: We don't know how to suffer. _____ 1

1. The night chaplain strides the halls. _____ 13

2. If I can't kill, then I can't heal. _____ 23

3. With each step we become a little more transparent. ____ 35

4. I just want to go home. _____ 43

5. He has resolved the question of life and death. _____ 61

6. Cassandra and Alexander the Great. _____ 71

7. Defeated, decisively, by constantly greater beings. ____ 89

8. Nothing special. We get them all the time. _____ 111

9. I have lost so much in my life. _____ 125

10. Seeing the pebbles clearly on the bottom. _____ 139

11. Oh, is that so? _____ 149

12. Please take care of me. _____ 167

13. I am not an animal! _____ 175

14. How does the music do that? _____ 185

Acknowledgements _____ 197

About the author _____ 201

Foreword

When I was in my second year as a faculty member four decades ago, I came to realize that I had a great deal of work to do on myself if I was going to be effective as a teacher of others. Family medicine has always embraced the behavioral sciences as an essential element of doctoring. But my medical model training equated behavioral science with psychiatry, and psychiatry, even 50 years ago, was more about biological models and pharmaceuticals than about what I was discovering that a family doctor needed to learn.

In the hospital, I came across a young pastor who was working there as part of his training to be a chaplain. My knowledge of chaplaincy was superficial, to say the least, mostly thinking of a priest being called to anoint the dying as a hedge against an eternity of suffering. I hadn't thought about chaplains as people who worked with the suffering of the living. But Tom told me about his clinical pastoral education course in Worcester and the challenging and intensive nature of his learning. I was jealous.

The medicine I had learned to that point was about physician agency, primarily diagnostic and therapeutic agency through machines, laboratories, and physical examination. Sometimes medicine felt like a mind game, trying to match a symptom with a diagnosis with a treatment. But even early in my career, I understood that the type of medicine my colleagues and I practiced was about doctoring where relationships matters most, where interventions are not pharmaceutical or surgical but, as the British psychoanalyst Michael Balint wrote, primarily concern the use and the misuse of the most commonly prescribed drug, the drug named "doctor".

I was fortunate to find two teachers who would guide me through the complex nature of relationships. One was a psychologist at Clark University who taught me how to formulate my questions about the doctor patient relationship in studies and reading that would train me about the scientific method applied to the daily work of family doctoring. The other was the chaplain, not a lot older than I was, who would talk regularly with me about his profound immersion into clinical pastoral education and how it taught him about preparing for his future work.

I hungered for a way to get the insights that he was getting into the nature of health and suffering and, through my psychologist professor/teacher, help meld the two disciplines of pastoral and medical education to create a safe space to process all the questions and challenges of doctoring and teaching. We started meeting early every Thursday morning in a hospital cafeteria in 1974. The meeting still goes on 43 years later. The model for presenting a case in that long-lived group was and is the narrative form used in clinical pastoral education.

In this wonderfully personal book about being inside that training all the time for three months, Gordon Greene helps many of us who don't know either the process or the goals learn about how they are framed in pastoral education. To use a phrase, particularly apt for Greene who is a Zen priest and a master swordsman, to learn what it is to "battle the invisible swordsman". While in Zen training, that battle is literal, those of us not from a Zen tradition can use that phrase as a metaphor to genuinely examine the struggles of our own lives.

Greene is a great storyteller and is courageous and not a little risky in letting us inside his own process of learning by being challenged and challenging himself in the important ways that clinical pastoral education demands. Demand is the operative word. No one gets a free pass.

It is clear that Greene was ready for this. Despite saying his interest was in "how a chaplain gets trained and employed in the Midwest", he did not enter training uninformed about the intensity and challenge it would require. After reading his deeply personal description of the program and its effects on him, I suspect that what appears to have been a casual interest on his part really was the full recognition that training would be a physical and emotional struggle with himself, both present and past.

I am often tempted to ask people who start on journeys "why now?" One of my more active professional roles at the moment is career counselling with colleagues and I ask them that question all the time and they often respond with feelings more than facts. If, prior to his beginning his chaplaincy training, I asked Gordon Greene, "why now" I suspect his answer would have been "I was ready to do battle."

Greene's Zen and sword training infuses his reflection on his pastoral education – he frequently uses the word "muscular" to describe the type of chaplaincy he is working toward, and surrounds it with physical metaphors of stance and breathing. In Genesis, Jacob wrestles all night with an Angel or, some interpret it, God, and is renamed Israel because he could not be defeated.

It occurred to me that Greene was wrestling – in his wonderful metaphor, battling the invisible swordsman – during the training he describes in his book. And if I asked him who he was wrestling with, who is the invisible swordsman, he would answer "suffering" but he also, throughout the book, would have to answer "myself".

There is much for us to learn from being along on Gordon Greene's struggles: humility, strength, compassion, frustration, anger and even about St. John of the Cross's "dark night of the soul."

The book at times feels like an intellectual tennis game: it goes back and forth from an objective presentation of a case of a patient encountered in the hospital or emergency room to a soul searching analysis of what the chaplain's role with this patient felt like and speculation about the underlying dynamics of the encounter.

Occasionally the ball deviates to the spiritual analysis and theory behind Greene's role as a Zen chaplain. In that process, we learn about the history and process of training in Zen, its various branches and traditions, and makes one want to learn the stance and breathing at its core. Since I suspect that most readers will not be familiar with those traditions, the book also serves as an introduction of Zen training as it applies to the care of self and others.

Clinical pastoral education is, after all, about understanding and applying spiritual methods to patient care – to the physical and spiritual suffering of people in pain.

In the end, Greene beautifully summarizes the understanding he has gained in a way that is really a prescription for health professionals as well as chaplains "To state it in the simplest terms, when I face suffering, I ease the suffering of those I face. The act of facing someone in anguish, in and of itself starts to ease that suffering."

One does not have to be in the health professions, though, to face someone in anguish. They are all around us, some more visible than others. The work of clinical pastoral education, then, can be applied to the work of family, friends, neighbors and society. As Pope Francis put it "The other has a face. The 'you' is always a real presence, a person to take care of." As Gordon Greene describes his training, it is a journey to the real presence of the other. But he also points out that, sometimes, the person to be taken care of is ourself.

John J. Frey III, MD
Emeritus Professor
Chairman, 1993 – 2006,
    Department of Family Medicine
        and Community Health
    University of Wisconsin School of Medicine
        and Public Health
President, 1998 – 1999,
    Society of Teachers of Family Medicine

Introduction:
We don't know how
to suffer.

I had just come off a 24-hour chaplain shift at Meriter Hospital in Madison, Wisconsin. After a long night spent with a patient and many of his family members, the morning's cold, rainy weather matched my mood. I felt raw and spent, empty.

The morning hand-off to the day team of chaplains began as it usually does, but when one of these colleagues asked me how I was doing, I started crying. My tears were no more than halfway down my cheek when the hospital on-call pager, still on my hip, went off, announcing a fresh emergency.

The beep of that pager pulled me out of my grief as I passed the call to the chaplain coming on duty. Someone was hurting. It was time for him to work. The moment for my own care had passed, as it does — day in, day out

— for busy nurses, physicians, and chaplains in an emergency room, an intensive care unit, a psychiatric ward.

I had cried over one of last night's patients: a middle-aged husband, father, son, and alcoholic. Brian was brought by ambulance to the hospital following a heavy bout of drinking that he must have known would kill him. Just one month before, he had been hospitalized with blood clots and had been on blood thinners since. Brian had been warned not to drink but now he was back. A CT scan showed more blood on his brain than the ER physician had ever seen before. This husband, father and son was now dead.

That night, my work as chaplain began with the patient's wife when she arrived with her husband at the emergency room. Over the next hour we were joined in Room 2 by his son, his wife's parents and three more relatives. With each new arrival, the stories of alcoholism in the family kept expanding. There were tales of relatives who got clean and stayed that way, but others who didn't and died young. Some lived with alcoholism well-masked, others wrecked every life they touched.

My pain was watching, hearing, how this disease washed through so many lives over so many generations, and how all this experience had not been enough to save the life of this man.

As a chaplain, my job is to ease suffering. Patient after patient, family after family, day after day. This "job" is shared by many: the medical staff in that emergency room or a social worker trying to place an elderly widower into a nursing home because he can no longer take care of himself at home. There is the person running a homeless shelter on a cold night in a big city, the journalist trying to convey the suffering in a refugee camp. There's a daughter caring for her mother as she lives out her days with Alzheimer's disease, and a parent trying to keep her teenaged son from cycling in and out of jail. How do these people learn to face human suffering? How do any of us?

My starting point is that for the most part we don't. We don't know how to suffer. We know how to avoid suffering. We may know how to shield ourselves from suffering or cope with suffering. And, many people have learned to survive suffering. But if you don't know how to suffer, your ability to help those who are suffering is limited.

Common responses when faced with suffering include detachment, distortion or immediate efforts to problem-solve. These strategies are rarely effective. But what works better? To answer that question, this book recounts a three-month internship in Clinical Pastoral Education (CPE), the training that introduced me to the work of hospital chaplains.

Long before entering that program, I had been a husband and father, and had spent years training in Zen Buddhism. I had become a priest, using my Zen training and life experience to teach medical students and physician residents how better to deal with their patients' suffering.

This experience means I began CPE already informed by decades of learning how to suffer and, therefore, how to face the suffering of others. But I didn't know how much I had yet to learn. CPE was difficult, intense, and one of the most exciting periods of learning in my life.

Out of that experience I was able to shape a muscular form of chaplaincy, a physical form of chaplaincy that treated it as manual labor. I use that phrase "manual labor" carefully, seeking to describe the kinds of strength and sensitivity needed to work effectively, both when things are calm and when things are out of control.

My need to learn to face suffering began in Honolulu when my youngest son was born. My wife Patricia's pregnancy had been a difficult one. But on the morning of Sam's birth I had not been particularly worried. We had a physician who we trusted completely and who had been a steady guide. And I had been present years earlier for the easy births of my son Alex and daughter Laura. In the hospital delivery room that morning with Patricia, there was just the immediacy of her breathing, and anticipation of seeing my new son.

But when Sam arrived into the hands of our doctor, he did not look like the newborns I had known. He was blue, not red or pink. There was no movement; he was a limp weight in the doctor's hands as he was carried to a cart set up with heating lamps and soft blankets. Sam was alive but slow to begin breathing.

My exhausted wife didn't yet know why she wasn't holding our baby. Patricia was saying, "Something's not right, something's not right." Her uterus had ruptured, and she was bleeding. A surgeon was evaluating her, preparing for emergency surgery.

Then someone in the room said, "Mr. Greene, we need to transport your son to Kapiolani." I was confused. Why go somewhere else? The Honolulu hospital for women and children he mentioned was fifteen minutes away. "Your son needs to go. Now. He'll get better care there. Do we have your permission?"

I had just learned that Patricia's surgery was successful when I received a phone call from an anxious, tired OB/GYN resident physician at Kapiolani Hospital, summoning me to the emergency room of the children's hospital. Upon my arrival, the physician said, "Mr. Greene, I need your permission to give your son an anti-seizure drug."

"OK. Why does Sam need that?"

"Well, children born with cerebral palsy often have seizures that are hard to control once they start. We use this drug to help prevent them from starting."

I had stopped listening after "cerebral palsy." I found myself, an ordained Buddhist priest, bargaining with the God of my childhood. "What do you need from me? I want Sam to love climbing in the Tetons the way I love climbing in the Tetons. How is that going to happen?"

During his three weeks in the neonatal intensive care unit Sam had no seizures or other serious complications. We cautiously brought him home to our tiny apartment in a quiet Honolulu neighborhood and visits to the pediatrician and the pediatric neurologist soon began. Having watched his erratic arm movements and felt his stiffness when we picked him up, on one visit Patricia said, "Something is not right." And Sam's neurologist answered, "He had a rough start, but now he is doing well. Everything is within normal limits."

I asked, "But what about that resident I talked to the day Sam was born? What about cerebral palsy?"

"He was just a resident. Nobody gets diagnosed with cerebral palsy at birth. Everything is within normal limits. Just relax and Sam will be fine."

Ten months later, everything was not within normal limits. Sam was not fine.

Our doctor broke the news. "I'm sorry to tell you that your son has a form of cerebral palsy. It's too soon to say exactly what kind, but there are many parents who have been able to love their children in this condition." Patricia recalls hearing, "You may want to consider the likelihood of placing your son in an institution."

All those months of feeling isolated, knowing something was wrong with Sam's health but only hearing that everything was "within normal limits." There had been no explanation of what "normal limits" meant or how they were measured. There were no attempts by Sam's physicians to explore our feelings of despair. As a result of that cold-hearted office encounter, our pediatrician and neurologist were fired that day. Take your normal limits and be damned.

Not long after learning that Sam's unusual muscle movements had a name, I was asked to apply for a position in the newly-formed Department of Family Medicine at the medical school at the University of Hawaii. I had no background in medicine, but the chairman of the department knew me as a Buddhist priest who had undergone intense training in a Zen monastery for three years.

When suggesting I apply, Dr. Takemoto-Gentile said, "We talk a lot about the art of medicine, and we know it in practice when we see it, but we have no idea how to teach it. See what you can do. You already seem to have the instincts for this art from your own Zen training."

This new job gave me a focus for the pain Patricia and I had experienced during her pregnancy and the months following Sam's birth. My mission was to teach medical students and residents how to better understand their patients — perhaps a child, or a mother in their care — and to heal them of suffering. This meant understanding their needs, their fears and, of course, their symptoms. But it also meant how to find what could be therapeutic in the relationship between physician and patient itself.

I wanted to teach skills that would have eased the pain that Patricia and I had so recently experienced. Heartfelt stuff and worthy goals, right? — but oh so naïve, I soon learned.

Wandering through the medical school curriculum, I was introduced to the tradition called "physician detachment." This phrase describes a physician's ability to separate themselves from their patients' suffering in order to maintain a necessary objectivity, supposedly allowing physicians to better draw upon their knowledge and experience.

Over the course of my life, as a patient I had encountered detachment across many medical encounters, but I had never heard it justified. Now that I was becoming part of the medical culture, I was curious. In one medical journal article I read, "The capacity to separate self from other is a key component of empathy; otherwise, the sight of another's pain can become paralyzing."

This "separation of self" violated everything I had learned as a Zen priest. It cemented in place a false dichotomy: that a physician must remain numb to a patient's suffering or become debilitated by it. Over years of Zen training, I had discovered a far different path. When faced with someone's suffering, that pain passes through you in such a way that you remain fully aware of all the sensations and emotions it evokes, but none of them stick. Your thinking, your words, your actions remain clear and efficient.

This ability is physical, visceral. It is not a belief or an abstract virtue. It is a physical phenomenon developed through refinement of one's breath and posture.

This refinement is a constant theme throughout this book, looking at the impact of breath and posture on both the person providing care to others as well as directly to those patients.

While these principles were continually being developed in my Zen training, they didn't come alive until one day during a week-long course for medical students in Tokyo. It was late July and hot and humid, with no breeze. I melted into the sound of cicadas as day after day, without relief, I walked between my hotel and the hospital. But one day, on one of those walks I realized that if I walked and breathed in a certain way, I didn't feel so incredibly hot.

I hadn't known it was possible until that moment. That I could alter my experience without changing anything in that swamp of air I was walking through.

I had witnessed some version of this same kind of optimization during my first visit to Israel several years ago, during the Second Intifada. Before arriving in Tel Aviv, I expected to find a certain degree of anxiety in everyone, living as they did in a setting where violence could suddenly erupt.

I found the opposite.

Everyone appeared relaxed as they walked the streets. I was confused until I recognized that this was a particular kind of relaxation. It considerably sharpened hearing and intuition. People were instinctively using breath and posture to ensure survival in dangerous conditions.

This focus on breath and posture relates as well to a second major theme of this book: most work is manual labor. In any job or profession, you need skills, knowledge and experience—concepts easily understood—but you also need your body.

This concept came alive for me when I was asked to develop a one-day workshop for a group of grade school teachers, introducing them to core principles of Zen Buddhism. Rather than lecturing about Buddhism as expected, for half the day I led them through exercises to help awaken awareness of breathing and posture.

We then shifted into role playing scenarios developed by them, recreating common classroom experiences. For example, in one scenario they tried to help students shift their attention from an hour's lessons in reading to an hour's lessons in math. We studied how the shift of the teacher's whole body influenced the ways in which their students made their shift.

Later, when I worked at the medical school, I applied this same kind of learning to students there. While trained how to prescribe antibiotics, they never learned how to properly stand when facing a patient. These future doctors may have heard it was good to place a hand on someone's shoulder when giving bad news, but nobody taught them the difference between an ordinary touch and a therapeutic touch.

One of my training techniques became known as the Knocking Exercise. As above, I told students that patients often have an animal instinct regarding the healing abilities of their physician, even before seeing them. Patients might judge this quality from the sound of footsteps in the hall or even the physician's knock on the examination room door.

To demonstrate this, I asked five student volunteers to leave the lecture hall and wait outside for my signal to re-enter the room. To those students still in the hall, I explained that each of the students outside was going to role-play the act of a physician knocking on the examination room door—in this case, the lecture hall door. They would each knock at 30-second intervals, walk in and sit down without saying anything. The job of the students in the hall would be to sit with their eyes closed, deciding at the sound of the knock if they felt the person about to enter was someone that could heal them.

The faces of the students sitting in the room clearly showed clear differences as they heard five distinct sets of knocking. Some of the knocks were warm in feeling, some cold and efficient, some hesitant, some confident.

The next year, we staged the same exercise for a new class of medical students. We started it the same way: five student volunteers leaving the lecture hall, students inside briefed, students outside briefed. There was a similar range of reactions as the first four students knocked and entered at 30-second intervals.

The fifth knock sent a chill down my spine. I saw a similar reaction in some student faces. And, I later heard of a similar reaction from faculty members observing this exercise. This fifth student was not one I knew well, but nothing especially stood out about her other than her spine-chilling knock.

Three weeks later, she asked to leave the medical school for medical reasons, later disclosed to be related to her mental health. She did not return to school. Somehow, her knock was diagnostic of a disturbed state of being. To my embarrassment, none of us as faculty acted upon our gut reaction that something was wrong and that she might need help.

My son Sam brought these themes alive for me. Without his difficult birth twenty-seven years ago, I doubt I would have taken the medical school position. Without that position, I most likely would not have trained as a hospital chaplain. Without working as a hospital chaplain, I would not have had as rich of an opportunity to test the breath and posture of my Zen training in the emergency settings found in emergency rooms, in intensive care units, in the rooms of dying patients.

Before the next chapters move the story into those hospital rooms, I'll report that Sam is continuing his research in theoretical chemistry after two years in Oxford as a Rhodes Scholar. If you met him, you would be swept up into an engaging conversation on any one of a dozen topics of current interest. And yes, a few years ago we did go hiking in the Tetons.

1.
The Night Chaplain strides the halls.

An intensive care unit nurse paged me around 5 a.m. The unit had just admitted a university student who had overdosed on a large amount of caffeine pills and had been driven by his roommate to the emergency room.

When I arrived at his ICU room, Evan was highly agitated, insisting on a broad interpretation of the patients' rights handout he had received in the emergency room, including his right to refuse care. My role was vague and unspecified by the nurses, but they certainly wanted me to calm Evan down or act as an intermediary to help them manage his demands. A hospital security officer also showed up; there was a feeling that Evan might need to be restrained.

He continued to challenge the nurses' instructions, forcing the nurses to ask Evan's permission for each new step critical for his care. He adapted the tactic of asking for five minutes alone with the chaplain first. Finding Evan to be well-educated I asked him what the philosopher Immanuel Kant might do if he found himself similarly restrained in a hospital. I know little of Kant, but my question sent Evan off on a wild ramble of ideas.

With time, Evan seemed to be calming down, though his nurses asked if I would stay with him until his medications kicked in. They really wanted him to fall asleep. I pulled up a chair and told him that I was interested in exploring the role of storytelling in chaplain work. I said I had stories I could tell him, but I would rather hear him tell a story, if he was so inclined.

Evan jumped at the chance, saying he wanted to tell me the story of the slave ship Amistad. I had only a vague understanding of this episode in American history and encouraged him to tell the story.

It was hard to follow as he laid out a tale with numerous dead ends and unrelated trajectories, but he tried with good heart to tell a coherent narrative as he grew sleepier and sleepier. Finally, sleep took over, and I was just able to show up in time for the 7:45 a.m. handoff to the day team of chaplains.

I worked as a night chaplain at Meriter Hospital, my first role in spiritual care for patients. I liked the drama. I liked my role in the drama. A physician friend enjoyed hearing my stories of patients from the middle of the night, saying they reminded him of the exhaustion and excitement from his own nights of residency training. He suggested that together we write a television series called "Night Chaplain," following a rugged chaplain into that dark night of the soul that seems to come when the hospital halls have been darkened and the only movement is the bobbing head of a ward clerk fighting off sleep.

As noble as that scenario might sound, there wasn't much spiritual care provided to that caffeinated Evan. I had been working more from instinct than training while helping to diffuse his agitation. His immediate needs had been expertly handled by the nurses and the security officer, but little was done to address his suffering. Why had Evan taken those caffeine pills in the first place?

This role as night chaplain began without much planning. I had moved with my family to Wisconsin from Hawaii, leaving behind my work with medical students in order to develop a Zen training temple. During my time in Hawaii, I had never met a chaplain, nor even heard of their work with patients, but instinct led me to explore how chaplains were trained and employed in Madison, home of the University of Wisconsin.

The CPE training program was based at a community hospital. Their full training program—a three-month internship, followed by a year-long residency—led to board certification as a chaplain. While that would have taken more time than I had available, they did have a Night Chaplain program more flexible in its requirements.

I made an appointment with Jeff Billerbeck, the director of the program. When we met in person, I was pleased by two things: he understood and valued the physicality of "presence" when providing patient care, and he also felt my experience as a Zen priest and a medical educator might be sufficient for the night chaplain role without the need for preliminary training. I would stay in the hospital one night every month, serving on call for whatever situations nurses or physicians felt required a chaplain.

During the days at this hospital, there were several full-time staff chaplains, as well as the chaplains training in the CPE program, but from 5:00 p.m. until 7:45 a.m. the following morning there was only one hospital chaplain covering the emergency room, intensive care unit, psychiatric ward, birthing suites and general care units.

It is hard to describe how fulfilling this job sounded to me. All those years at the medical school, talking about physicians themselves becoming therapeutic instruments, but only talking. Now I had the chance to be that instrument, to become that healing presence, to bring my Zen training into a life and death arena.

It took me back to the first time I had a taste of what it might mean to be a clinician. As a brand-new medical educator, I had spent several nights in Oahu's Wahiawa General Hospital, taking overnight calls with the Family Medicine residents so that I could better understand the nature of their training.

One memorable night, the on-call resident brought me to the small Emergency Room so I could meet the physician on service, Dr. Thomas, a man known as a good teacher. Dr. Thomas asked me to see a newly-arrived patient while he finished up with someone else.

"You don't understand. I'm the medical educator with the residency program, not a resident."

But Dr. Thomas had heard of me and my role in the department. "If you want to learn what we do, do it. Don't watch it."

There I was, in a small room with a large Samoan man who had badly cut his hand while fishing offshore that night. Two of his sons had been with him, had brought the boat in, and had driven him to the emergency room. The sons sat quietly as blood soaked through the towel wrapped around their father's hand, dripping on the floor beside the gurney. I think that the sum total of my work with that patient was to say, "Dr. Thomas will be in to take care of you in a minute." Then I too sat there silently.

That felt useless, but Dr. Thomas thanked me for my help once he had sewn up the wound. And I started to feel a kind of glow. If the doctor thanked me, I must have provided care. It sounds juvenile in hindsight but having interviewed dozens of applicants to medical school in Hawaii, I now recognize how many times I heard applicants describe a similar experience, however trivial, when they truly felt they had provided care. That was all the spark it took to ignite the hard, slow process to apply to medical school. With a fair degree of delusion, I too felt like a medical student.

I lay out this memory, fifteen years before I began my work as a night chaplain, to illustrate the hunger I brought to the role. I badly wanted to have professional standing in a setting where human tragedies unfolded. No one had asked me to do that in my role as a medical educator. And no one had asked me to do that in my role as a Zen priest.

No one had said, "Gordon," or "Dr. Greene," my academic title, or "Reverend Greene, get in there and take care of Mrs. Suzuki in Room 8."

In this community hospital, it was different. I was briefed by the day-time chaplains at 4:45 p.m. Then I strapped on the on-call pager and began seeing patients that the day team had not yet been able to. All the time, I waited for the pager to signal I needed to respond to an urgent need. By protocol at this hospital, "urgent need" meant any patient coming into the emergency room with a suspected stroke or heart attack, any patient coming in with a "Level 2 trauma," such as a fall or a minor automobile accident or gunshot wound, any patient about to die, and any patient who had stopped breathing or whose heart stopped.

My proscribed role for these urgent pages was more to help any family members who might be present, or who should be called in, rather than to help the patients. But I gave myself latitude, learning how to be present to any patient without disrupting any emergency medical care being provided.

Any nurse or physician could also call for my help when they felt a chaplain would be useful to a patient.

This might be an elderly woman, unable to sleep, crying because of fear or loneliness. Or a young man making frequent and unnecessary demands of the nurses. Often there were no easy medical solutions.

For example, Theodore's wife had been admitted to one of the general wards a few days earlier with a seemingly benign blood chemistry imbalance. She was now having emergency surgery to insert a heart pacemaker. Theodore was a stoic 80-year-old whose wife was now in a life-threatening condition. We had already spent 30 minutes together, as his wife was being resuscitated following an unexpected Code Blue. She was now in the catheterization laboratory and it was time to wait for the results.

I asked a few minor questions, mostly just to see how Theodore was feeling. I got one-word answers and nothing more. I decided to wait without talking. Five minutes, no talking. Ten minutes, no talking.

Somewhere just before twenty minutes had gone by, Theodore started to talk. With passion, with detail. About their early life together. About their children. About his heart surgery several years earlier. About fears for his wife.

What I learned with Theodore was the power of silence, but not just any silence. An open silence, a working silence, a visceral, purposeful silence, in which words are welcome but not necessary.

This work was highly meaningful to me, but I was only on duty as a night chaplain once a month. It was not enough. I wondered if I could bring the same degree of motivation, of creativity, and of caring if I had to face patients every day. I had doubts. Maybe I'm not really as good at this work as I think I am. But I had an intense hunger to learn more, so I applied for the formal chaplain training program.

Going into the interview, I had thought my admission to the program would be easily accepted after a thoughtful discussion of why I felt chaplaincy training would be interesting. Instead, I found myself quickly engaged in a forceful conversation with no sense of whether or not I was anywhere close to being accepted into the program. This was a tough crowd.

The most seasoned chaplain asked: "What can you tell us about the role of emotion in Buddhism?"

I answered, "I can't speak for all of Buddhism. I really only know my own lineage of Zen Buddhism, namely Rinzai Zen. There are two things I would say. The first is that emotions are like waves on the ocean, a disturbed surface underlain by a deep column of water with slow and certain long-term currents. Our training is to move with that deeper water and to not be caught up in the waves on the surface..."

My interviewer interrupted. "Bullshit! What are your emotions right now?"

"I'm feeling like I'm in the midst of a fight. And that sensation comes from my heart rate, my breathing, and from the kind of vision I am experiencing right now. And that actually is the second thing I wanted to say about emotion. For any given emotion, there are physical sensations that produce it. Emotion is not in my head as an idea, but it is a set of feelings in my body. Those sensations are what I have been trained to readily recognize, though I don't necessarily state the associated emotion. That would be an unnecessary abstraction from the sensation. What else am I feeling? I feel surprised that my approach to my chaplain work is being challenged rather than explored. Is there only one way to be a chaplain?"

The social worker answered, "I don't think you understand the work of a chaplain. What do you think you do as a chaplain?"

Without thought, I said, "Take away fear."

There was no answer from the group. I wondered why Jeff, the director of the chaplain training program, wasn't speaking up more. Strange, because he had been very encouraging when I said I would like to apply.

The next question was, "Do you have a problem with respect for Jeff or [the assistant director] Chuck?" Perhaps because I had been a faculty member at a medical school, they thought I had an exalted opinion of myself.

Answering this question was easy. In my first meeting with Jeff, he had said that he had two primary interests in his work as the Director of Spiritual Care for this hospital: evidence-based chaplaincy, and something he called the "presence" of a chaplain. Like me, Jeff felt the work was not about being nice to people. It was about helping them heal faster.

As for "presence," the word that summarizes the impact of skilled non-verbal communication, including body language—was home ground for me as a Zen priest. I had been pleased to find someone in a position of authority in a hospital acknowledge this as a trainable skill. I felt this had been one reason that Jeff was so supportive of my application—because I already knew and could demonstrate "presence."

As for my relationship with Chuck, I told a story to the interview team about coming off night chaplain service one morning when Chuck asked me how I was doing. Whatever your religion or belief, if you have ever been asked that question by a priest (and Chuck is an Episcopalian priest), it can come with a deeper sense of inquiry than what might happen when a friend or colleague asks the same question.

That morning with Chuck, I described the struggles my wife was having as her father was dying, which brought unexpected tears. I told my interviewers that I respected anyone who could evoke those in me with just a simple question.

The interview ended with the oldest chaplain saying, "Well, I'm not sure what to predict about your training. but I think you are going to have a very interesting time."

Quite prophetic.

2.
If I can't kill,
then I can't heal.

As my colleagues and I were getting to know each other during an afternoon seminar in the first week of CPE training, I played a favorite recording of a truck-driving song for them. There was something about Taj Mahal singing "Six Days on the Road" that described me better than I could describe myself. It wasn't the lyrics so much as it was an exuberant "baby, baby, baby" Taj Mahal snuck into a verse that captured the abundance of happiness he felt as he was about to see his woman again. The lyrics as written, the notes as played, could not contain that degree of happiness. He needed that "baby, baby, baby" and so did I.

I described how my grandmother schooled me early in my life in what she called the "minor epiphanies" of her own life, pointing to moments she had experiences beyond the ordinary and rational. I said that my own life felt "ecstatic," not sure what I meant to say with that word but feeling a bursting of my own ordinary and rational as we began our training.

This may have been a part of me long-buried, a part that a grade-school teacher once told my mother was exciting to see but hard to deal with. That teacher said she had never seen such a drive to learn. Starting my CPE training, I felt that force within me again being unleashed.

The first week we began our training's basic rhythm: clinical work with patients, small group learning with my CPE colleagues, reflective writing, and one-on-one supervision with Jeff. And then repeat.

The early days of group work included a fair amount of storytelling: short and quick versions of who we were, then longer narratives. It quickly became clear that the four of us in training were all highly motivated to learn.

Linda and Scott had more than two decades of service as pastors to specific congregations, with each of them recently dismissed from their positions for reasons not easily understood. Each had experienced their discharge as a painful challenge to their sense of identity, and they wanted to use a full year of chaplain training to explore the meaning of healing, for themselves and others.

Collin was much younger, having just finished his training at Harvard Divinity School. He was back in the Midwest, close to the home of his youth out in the country, very close to where I live. He was also compelled to understand the nature of healing. Like the other two, he was called a "resident," meaning he would be training in clinical pastoral education for a full year.

I was an intern, meaning that I would be training fulltime for just the first quarter of their year. Usually, interns train with other interns, with only minor overlap with the residency training, but our supervisor Jeff felt that the four of us would blend well and allowed me to join them.

Jeff Billerbeck was the director of clinical pastoral education, working in that role for more than two decades, providing a powerful and effective model of quiet spiritual care and chaplain trainee supervision.

With Jeff, his means of supervision did not so much involve telling anyone what to do. Instead, he showed a personal vulnerability, a willingness to share his own experiences, including fears, doubts and longings. This helped me discover my own.

During the five weekdays, we had three half-days of small group teaching, one hour of one-on-one time with Jeff as supervisor, a medical team meeting to review the course of treatment and healing for patients who had been hospitalized for more than two weeks, and our pastoral care duties on our assigned units. Our days began at 7:45 a.m., with the hand-off from the night chaplain and continued until 4:45 p.m. when we briefed the night chaplain coming on service.

On the weekends we took turns providing 24-hour coverage. During that time, we covered the entire hospital, working alone just as I had during my work as a night chaplain.

Beyond all this, we were writing about ourselves and our patients in a broad range of formats, producing twelve to fifteen thousand words per week.

These three months of encounters with patients and with my CPE supervisor and colleagues dramatically changed how I faced suffering. Who was I at this point beyond my identity as a 61-year-old man and Zen teacher struggling to build a Zen training center? I was also a husband, struggling to find my voice in a marriage rife with many damaged channels of communication with my wife Patricia. And I was working to rebuild a close relationship with my son Alex and daughter Laura from my first marriage— both adults now, struggling in their own marriages.

By this time, my youngest child Sam was a sophomore at the University of Chicago, deepening his interest in theoretical chemistry. It seemed to be the tool with which he wanted to help address the complex issues of climate change, a subject he became focused on during early school years in Hawaii. The impact of his cerebral palsy showed in the awkwardness of his walking and his speech but hadn't touched his ability to think and write clearly.

But saying such things so matter-of-factly doesn't do justice to the many struggles Sam had been making for many years, using his physical therapy, his occupational therapy, and his speech therapy as tools to help him appear as normal as possible.

Similarly, for my wife Patricia and myself, we wanted him to have that sense as well. We had not been part of support groups for parents of children with cerebral palsy. We didn't seek out families with members who had cerebral palsy. During his childhood, we were aggressive in seeking medical care that would help Sam's walking. But by the time Sam was nineteen years old, we were all living something of a double life, profoundly aware of the daily impact of the damage to his neuromuscular system, but also pretending that it didn't matter.

It is fair to say that my need to learn to face suffering that had begun decades before had something of a double nature. I easily focused on teaching about this as a medical school faculty member. It was easy to focus on this as a Zen teacher. But other than facing suffering in my own family and with the patients that I had seen during my one night each month as a night chaplain, I didn't really know what I was talking about.

That admission lay beneath another answer to the question of "Who am I?" Because I liked my identity as a teacher of medical students and my title as a Zen teacher, I was proud, arrogant, self-assured, ready for anything. This was the person Jeff and the others interviewing me for admission to CPE were perhaps worried about. This was also the person about to come face to face with that identity and learn how poorly it served him or those he sought to serve.

I began my formal training on August 31. The first week was filled with patient encounters, orientation meetings, and small group sessions so that we four CPE colleagues could get to know each other. I'd had self-confidence working as a night chaplain, but felt like a true beginner in this work, awkward with patients and hesitant with medical staff.

My first chance to reflect on my work came in the first of my weekly one-on-one supervisor meetings with Jeff. The format was open-ended, beginning with his question, "What would you like to talk about?"

This was my first attempt to pick up the question asked of me during my interview for the CPE program: "What is the role of emotion in Buddhism?" I was starting to recognize that emotions may not be something that exists only within me. For those experiences to be considered emotions, rather than something sensory or visceral, perhaps they must be shared, experienced by another.

In this sense, I was starting to experience emotion as the natural language of human beings. But when expressed that way, it sounds like something exchanged between two objects, and that is not what I mean. It is more that this thing we call "emotion" is an emergent property that arises when we are in a state in which the ordinary barriers between self and other starts to dissolve. In other words, it is not a question of my sense of aliveness or enlargement. It is more the sense of aliveness or enlargement. Awkwardly expressed, but this is how I learn. At least say something and then see where that leads.

In our next small group meeting, the four of us shared our learning objectives for the next three months. I found it helpful to state an objective but also to describe how I would work to meet that objective, and what an objective measure of accomplishment might look like. How would I know I had succeeded?

For example, one of my objectives was to "Develop awareness of my senses in my pastoral relationship to patients, families and staff." My method for doing that would be to, at least once a day, write a short description of my sensory experiences when working with a patient. My progress in deepening that sensory awareness would be evaluated by my colleagues when I made occasional case presentations in future small group sessions.

I also had an objective to "Explore the question 'What is healing?'—so as to deepen my understanding of the Buddhist perspective on the alleviation of suffering."

Over the next three months, this goal became a focus. Not just the "What is healing?" but "Who is healing?" and "Who is being healed?" I was not satisfied with the common view of chaplains as people who simply bring comfort to patients. Most likely because of my years working already with medical students, I felt called to heal and not just comfort, even though I wasn't clear what this meant.

I received reinforcement for this goal within chaplaincy when members of our group read a short book by Paul Pruyser called The Minister as Diagnostician. Pruyser described diagnostic categories that he felt clergy should be trained to evaluate in the spiritual care of patients and to then treat. This was the language also used to train medical students: you diagnose, then you treat.

For example, one diagnostic category is "awareness of the Holy" or "open to transcendence." In Pruyser's way of thinking, a patient who has this awareness or openness is healthy, whereas one who does not may be suffering. Treatment then becomes the work of exploring how a patient may reconnect with their own sense of spirituality. This was a more muscular view of the work of chaplains and it aligned with the work of a Zen priest—we heal duality—but that phrase was more of an abstraction for me than a nuanced sense of technique. I wanted to explore the "how" of healing duality and Pruyser's book offered me permission to do that.

At my second weekly supervisory meeting with Jeff, I asked for feedback about my work in group. Jeff said that he liked my energy and enthusiasm, but we discussed an interaction with the palliative care team in which I made them uncomfortable. Jeff said, "There is enthusiasm and then there is over-enthusiasm"—and I am more prone to the latter than I realized.

The most significant part of the discussion came when I said, with a lot of hesitation, that I feel the potential for me to be "dangerous" in human interactions. In a Zen context, that is not necessarily a bad thing. I said this may arise from not fearing death. But Jeff's immediate challenge was "What about the death of a relationship?

That is the risk you take with your intensity."

Jeff reminded me of a comment I made not long after meeting him: "If I can't kill, then I can't heal." But the opposite must be equally true, "If I can't heal, then I must not kill." I thought I understood this basic Buddhist resolution of the duality of life and death, but not so. I was in an arena where healing and death are more immediate and thus more sharply in focus.

Two weeks into my training and I was already feeling devastated. Actually, "cracked open" better describes my state at the time. I was now staring at the damage I had done to my relationships with my two children from my first marriage. Though painful, that "cracked open" was a helpful sensation. On some level, that is why I came into CPE in the first place, even though I couldn't articulate that in my application. Zen training is a hammer on a black walnut, a way to crack open the shell of duality. Here that hammer was again.

To better explain that quality of danger in human interactions I'll recount a 17th century story based on an encounter between the Shogun of Japan, the swordmaster to the Shogun, and the great Zen teacher, Takuan Zenji.

It started when Shogun Iemitsu, master swordsman Yagyu, and Takuan were admiring an unusual gift to the Shogun: a caged but wild tiger. The Shogun asked Yagyu to demonstrate the manner in which he would face a dangerous opponent by approaching the tiger and stroking its head. Agreeing, Yagyu entered the cage. Holding just a fan before him as if it were a sword, Yagyu entered the cage and slowly advanced. The tiger growled but did not move as Yagyu placed his hand on its head. Slowly the swordsman retreated, leaving the cage drenched in sweat.

The Shogun then turned to Takuan and asked, "Has Zen anything else to show?" Unlike Yagyu, Takuan ran as easily into the cage as a young boy enjoying a meadow in early summer. Facing the tiger, he held his palm out to the tiger which sniffed and then licked his hand. With that, Takuan lightly touched its head, then turned and came out of the cage as easily as he went in. The story goes that Shogun's only comment was, "After all, our way of the sword cannot compete with Zen."

My ability to face suffering was akin to Yagyu approaching that tiger. There is a form of whole-body concentration that one learns in Zen training that has a quality of "no openings," meaning no place of vulnerability. If you've ever watched a cat stalk a bird in tall grass, you've seen something like this concentration. I was proud of this ability in myself. And somehow proud that it felt dangerous to people when they encountered this outside my familiar world of Zen and swordsmanship. But I was no Takuan, able to heal when faced with danger.

Coming into my CPE training as I did, hungry to learn, I brought in the association I already had between learning and risk. The more the risk, the more the learning. To the degree I was conscious of this association I felt justified in announcing to my small group that I liked "going all-out" in my learning, that I didn't need rules to guard my safety. But I wasn't recognizing how the others most likely felt differently.

And what is that phrase, "If I can't kill, then I can't heal"? It is hard for me to read my own untested pronouncements here. I'm not a physician and I have never been in combat, so this is me spouting theory un-tempered by experience. But I have to be honest and this ideal is something I carried inside myself. For better or for worse, it was part of me going into my CPE training.

This conviction came out of my early days as a family medicine residency program faculty member. There was a resident that was part of the residency training program whom we now felt should not graduate. This resident had a mix of personal and professional issues that they seemed unable to correct, despite a year's effort. It was time to release them from the program. Faculty members had carefully established clear criteria for completion of each rotation in the program, and these had not been met by this resident.

Given this, I was surprised how difficult it was for my physician colleagues to act. Certainly, we all were concerned about the consequences of graduating a family medicine physician that might compromise patient safety, but it was nevertheless still hard for my colleagues.

For these reasons, I became the "prosecuting attorney" in carrying out the dismissal hearings established by policy. In doing so, I felt that my colleagues were one-sided in their abilities. They were able to heal when it came to patients, but not able to "kill" when it came to dismiss a resident from the program.

In Jeff's terms, that dismissal was the "death of a relationship," and that was acceptable to me. However, when Jeff spoke during our supervisory session, I was not thinking of the relationship with that resident, but the many others in my life that felt broken. A sword cut can be clean and liberating but it can also make a mangled and bloody mess. I was feeling relationships that had ended as a mess.

3.

With each step we become a little more transparent.

Our CPE group's first written assignment was to "Choose a literary, biblical or mythical character with whom you identify and who reflects yourself. Focus on the feelings of this character as you imagine them in their particular life situation...Allow yourself freedom to project yourself into the character you have chosen."

I started the assignment by imagining myself as a young Kobo Daishi, a historical figure in Japanese Buddhism. After graduating from college, I had walked a thousand-mile pilgrimage on the Japanese island of Shikoku. Established centuries ago, the walk linked a number of temples and training sites associated with Kobo Daishi's life. That pilgrimage marked my first significant training in Buddhism, and I wanted to recapture some of that experience in my essay.

I worked on my Kobo Daishi essay for several days, but it never came alive. On the morning of the day I was to present my piece to my group, I felt uninspired, like I was just going through the motions. I didn't truly feel a meaningful connection to Kobo Daishi.

Over the one-hour lunch break before the group met, I decided to write as a literary character with whom I actually did identify: Peter Lake, the protagonist in Mark Helprin's novel, Winter's Tale.

The theme of the novel is Peter's effort to stop time and bring back the dead, and the book's style is magical realism. The settings and characters are ones any of us could recognize if we were visiting New York City, but in the novel, at the slightest provocation, the most ordinary of objects or people become quite extraordinary. That was the same exhilarating feeling I had while training in this community hospital. Sometimes a piece of writing feels as if it were done in just one breath. And that was true for this one:

Projective Character Study

Peter Lake is now a chaplain in training, walking down the staircase from the main lobby that goes to the back entrance of the Emergency Department. As he arrives at the ground floor, he sees a young physician, glasses and dark hair, opening the metal gate that prevents access from the ground floor to the hospital's lower levels.

Now, shifting the narrative to Peter's voice: I had heard that there was another unit of the hospital on a basement floor below the Emergency Department but knew nothing about it. Suddenly here was someone coming up from that basement floor. The unit I had heard of must actually exist, and I had to see it. But my ordinary duties continued and there was no chance that day.

But there came a Saturday when I was on 24-hour call at the hospital. All was calm: my patients seemed at some level of ease, and my two pages that day had been for patients who needed help but were not in crisis. It was late afternoon when I headed for that staircase, descending, opening the gate I had thought impassable. I went down one more flight of stairs.

The stairway door opened into a grove of white oaks. It looked to be a woodland savanna, with wide swaths of grasses between the trees. There were also small cabins scattered about the grove. And nurses, physicians, lab techs, walking about in their familiar garb but far from their familiar habitats.

A nurse recognized my gait as that of a chaplain and motioned me into a cabin. Here was a patient, her face showing the wrinkled strains of someone ill and freshly arrived in her search for care. She was resting in a chair as the nurse bought out samples of cloth: silk, linen, some were coarser, some were finer.

With each one, she invited the patient to touch it as she closed her eyes. The nurse observed what passed through this patient as she felt the cloth. And then there was a shift in the atmosphere of the room. The nurse told me, "This is how we choose bed linens for this woman while she is with us on this unit."

I stopped at another cabin when I overheard a conversation about food. A nurse with a newly arrived patient was asking for childhood memories of favorite meals or foods. Maybe a squash and sage soup that was served when the weather turned cool in the fall. Maybe a cookie in the oven near Christmas time. Or a peach, the first mouthful on a hot July day, mid-day when the air has gone still and all there is to existence is the heat and the sweet juice coming down your chin.

This nurse told me, "This is how we know what smells should come in the window throughout the day."

I moved onto a cabin where the patient was seated on a porch swing. Standing before it, the nurse was pushing the swing slowly at first, but then faster and faster. Watching the patient's face intently, there came a moment when she saw a broad smile and a slight relaxing of her patient's body. "Now we know how to move this patient's bed at night, matching the way his mother rocked him in her lap that evening in May as they watched the full moon rise, waiting for his father to come up the sidewalk."

As I left this cabin, I heard music in the distance: a cello playing the theme from Kitaro's "Silk Road." Oh, how that drew me to find the source, but I should have known who it was. There was a beautiful woman, hair like spun gold, a woman who had appeared at magical moments throughout my life, now playing her old companion, a cello made long ago in a workshop near Cremona.

And the sounds, the notes... As she played, it slowly brought into reality a caravan of travelers crossing the Gobi Desert. There were proud horsemen and sultry women and fat traders in the party and ragged monks toward the back who were carrying litters with people lying on them.

I realized that I was one of these monks, and the load we carried was that of the clinic patients from the grove of white oaks. And all of them were being transported to the majestic rhythm of that cello, each note carrying us forward to the night's oasis, still some distance ahead.

For all of us, patients and travelers alike, with each step we became more transparent, more of the sandstone and the sky showing through us. With each pulse of a step, each pulse of a note, we became more transparent. And our breathing became longer and deeper, closer and closer to becoming the wind that had begun to stir as the first hints of dusk came on.

You couldn't tell when it happened, but at a

certain moment, if you had looked away and now looked back, all of us, camels, horsemen, monks, dogs, dissolved into sandstone and sky and air. Yet still you could still hear the cello, and all had been healed.

Our habit in group was to take turns reading our essays aloud and then spending time discussing them. This discussion in particular helped me become conscious of values surrounding healing that I had not been aware of, certainly not while writing in such a rush.

I don't have Helprin's prose style, but felt that I had, like he does, written a kind of love story even if I cannot answer "Love of what?" It did illustrate how much I value the role of the senses in healing. That porch swing brought out such longing ...to be held, to be rocked.

"...and all had been healed." In some way, my closing line expressed an answer to one of my learning goals: What is healing? There is love, there is rhythm, there are senses, and there is no healer to be found.

It is a strange phrase, "no healer to be found," and I'll be wrestling with it throughout this book. On one level it refers to an effective softening of the ego, an act that allows more of the patient to be heard and seen. When fewer of the healer's normal filters are in place, there is clearer perception of what is needed and thus a richer form of healing.

The next day I had my third weekly supervisory conference with Jeff: a rich and deep conversation. My notes written afterwards capture the sensation of being in the discussion. We were talking about my training with a sword and the kind of dangerous atmosphere Yagyu created as he approach the tiger.

Thinking of last week's conference, I recognize that sheathing the sword diminishes none of the intensity that I crave. By making the conscious choice of sheathing the sword, I gain the freedom to use it appropriately. Nothing is lost, freedom is gained. So, the feeling becomes one of release, happiness, depth.

I went on to describe how I am drawn to patients with difficult lives—not just medically but in a "train wreck" of a life. What does this say about me? A positive interpretation would be that I am drawn to lives of clarity—no matter what the circumstances, these are lives lived without a veneer. Somehow it is easy to feel their humanity shining through, and that makes me feel alive.

Jeff said that I had a gift for listening in these settings and that I should cultivate that gift. I described an ability to listen without judgment and he suggested that I watch for those moments when I "pull up the reins"— meaning, something got to me, disturbed me—and then I should ask myself, "What was that?" Good idea.

Also discussed the strength and power available with intensity, but Jeff suggested that I look deep for moments of helplessness and despair. I described myself as always having a "plan B"—you'll never get me backed into a corner. But I can see how ultimately, a life lived that way has limits. If I can let in helplessness as it happens, I'll be better able to enter a patient's despair. I feel a freedom in knowing this. My face is relaxing as I think of this part of the conversation.

Finally, I described the highest level of swordsmanship—the stance called happo biraki in Japanese, translated as "open on all sides," meaning no conscious defense because there is nothing left of the Self to defend.

Of note here is a return to the imagery of a sword. I spoke earlier about Yagyu's approach to the tiger, holding his fan with the same intensity and focus he would have been if holding a sword. In this sense, Yagyu was not "open on all sides" as he approached the tiger. But Takuan, extending his hand to the tiger for a sniff, was. That is why the shogun acknowledged the wondrous quality of Takuan's approach.

When Jeff began asking me to look within for helplessness and despair, at the time these were qualities I held in disdain. Even if I could understand their importance in the lives of my patients, I couldn't acknowledge their importance for myself. That was to come later, from an unexpected direction.

4.
I just want to go home.

Three weeks into my training, and it felt like three months. One of the core training methods for clinical pastoral education was reflection, and already that felt like a relentless activity: reflection on patients, on myself, and on my colleagues.

To show how dominant this constant reflection had become, here is a conversation with one of my patients, an unmarried elderly gentleman called Mr. Peterson. At the time this conversation took place, he had been in the hospital for several days, with a condition not yet fully understood. I've labeled and numbered each part of the conversation, with my words as chaplain labeled "C" and the patient's words labeled "P."

C1: Hi, Mr. Peterson, do you remember me from two days ago? I'm Gordon, the chaplain who was visiting with you then.

P1: I'm glad to see you [said with a weak smile]. How have you been?

C2: I've been fine, but I have missed talking with you. How have you been doing?

P2: Well, not bad, I suppose. But I'm still troubled by all the things going on. But there will be people there this week and they should get things taken care of in a few weeks. The toilet... the microwave... [I thought at first Mr. Peterson was talking about his health condition but then realized he was speaking about his house, the one he had lived in for the past 53 years. This house and its maintenance problems had been a significant topic of conversation during our previous visit.]

C3: I'd like to hear more about this, but first please tell me about you. How are you feeling now?

P3: Well, they seem to be able to control the fever, but they don't know what is causing it yet. [He still has his weak but genuine smile and his voice is getting a little bit stronger.]

C4: OK... [said in a neutral tone. My thoughts are drifting a bit at this point. Why don't they know where this fever is coming from? He has had so many tests already. Why doesn't he appear more concerned about this? He is *more worried about his house than about his health...]*

P4: *I'm hoping I can leave this weekend. I'm going back to Fenmore [a skilled nursing facility where he had been recuperating from his previous hospitalization] so I can get my strength back.*

C5: *I'm glad you have so many people here helping you.*

P5: *I'm supposed to have an x-ray today, so I haven't had any food yet.*

C6: *That must be difficult.*

P6: *Oh, not really. I've only had one meal in the past two and a half days. [Really?] I don't really know what they've been doing, but all kinds of stuff. They take me here; they take me there...lots of stuff. [Still that weak smile and it is starting to feel a bit spooky. He really doesn't seem all that concerned with what's going on for him. He seems basically detached from his medical treatment and his medical condition.]*

[...a long pause...his smile is gone, and his eyes are a bit unfocused now...]

P7: *God, I can't stand much more of this... [said slowly and with a deep kind of resignation.]*

C7: *I'm sorry...*

P8: *I am so tired. [Mr. Peterson's eyes have gone half-closed.]*

C8: *What kind of tired?*

P9: *I just want to go home...*

C9: *I want that for you too. That place has been your life.*

P10: *Yes, it has. [said slowly, but his eyes light up a bit at this comment.] I have been praying...*

C10: *Well, I'd like for you to get some rest. But how about this? I do love listening to your voice and have a request: would you say the Lord's Prayer with me before I go?*

P11: *Sure.*

C/P: *Our father...*

P12: *You have been so good to me, everybody here has. You have such a kind face.*

C12: *Thank you. I've enjoyed spending time with you and hearing about your life. I won't be here this weekend so if you do go to Fenmore, I'm going to have to say my goodbyes now. Please take care of yourself and get back to that home that you love.*

P13: *Thank you. Please keep doing your good work. [said with sincerity. His face has softened during these last few minutes of talking.]*

C13: *Goodbye. [I'm feeling sad but also full of some kind of love (?) as I say this. I feel that I have seen him whole.]*

P14: *Goodbye.*

Capturing dialogue, setting it into context, and then reflecting on it all is part of a "verbatim," and is one of the core training methods for chaplain training. The verbatim centers on the words of an encounter with a patient, or a patient's family, or one of the medical staff, then analyzes this interaction in different ways.

Like psychologists and psychiatrists, chaplains need a high degree of self-awareness during any given encounter, an expectation also familiar to anyone training in Zen. The verbatim format acknowledges that there cannot be an objective description of a patient without also including descriptions of those interacting with this patient, as well as descriptions of the environment in which the interaction took place.

During the fifteen years I had spent in medical education, focusing on how to make the encounter itself between a physician and a patient be therapeutic, I had never seen anything like this form of analysis. It seemed so logical, so necessary, so efficient that I wondered why I had never heard of it before. To me, it became such a profound training device that, if I had the power, I would mandate its use in medical school curriculum during all four years of medical training.

Here's the rest of the first verbatim I wrote, following a standardized format:

Information about the patient:
Ministry Setting*: Unit 6 Tower*
Minister*: Gordon Greene*
Patient visit Number/ Length of Visit*: 3rd visit, 60 min*

Patient Age: *85*
Sex: *Male*
Patient Marital Status/ Number of Children:
never married, no children
Patient Religious Preference: *Lutheran*
Patient Admitting Diagnosis: *"acute fever and sepsis"*

Additional Factual Information:
Mr. Peterson, an 85 y.o. male nursing home patient with a history of non-oxygen dependent COPD, seizure disorder, chronic lower extremity edema with recent hospitalization, here for cellulitis and then hospitalization for pneumonia, who presents to the ER for a fever of 102 at the nursing home. The patient is a poor historian. He denies pain or any problems. He says he feels fine."

We will return to this physician's comment that this patient is a "poor historian." Here is what was listed for his known medical problems: hypertension, chronic lower extremity edema, obesity, tobacco abuse ("ongoing and severe"), COPD, hyponatremia, seizure disorder, pneumonia (recent hospitalization), cellulitis (recent hospitalization), urinary frequency, GERD, history of alcoholism, rheumatoid arthritis.

Social history upon admission includes, "Mr. Peterson has been living at Fenmore since these most recent hospitalizations, but prior to this was living independently with the help of outside assistance. He is wheelchair-bound." He was referred to the palliative care team because it was felt that he might not fully understand the serious state of his overall health. He would say, "Oh, I simply have a fever and as soon as I get better, I am going home." If a discussion about his more serious underlying problems is begun, Mr. Peterson deflects the questions. This is another expression of his status as a "poor historian."

I had visited with Mr. Peterson two previous times. During these I had learned more about his childhood, his parents, his work as an insurance salesman. He indeed had the persona of an insurance salesman: warm, interested in me, easy going. When asked if he had ever been married, Mr. Peterson talked about the effects of his alcoholism: it seems to have ruined his relationships with several women and had taken over his life before he joined Alcoholics Anonymous.

Mr. Peterson was raised a Lutheran but seems to have left his faith once he began drinking heavily. Asked about his faith now, he answered simply "AA." Asked about his God, he said, "The one I met in AA." He is also scheduled to have cataract surgery in about a month's time.

Plans:

My plan for this encounter with Mr. Peterson was to try to better understand the comment of the emergency physician who first saw him—"The patient is a poor historian"—and the comment heard during the palliative care rounds—"This guy is in denial." These comments suggest that Mr. Peterson is not playing by the rules of proper healthcare. Why not?

When I first heard these comments, my initial reaction was to prove the physician wrong. I thought that perhaps I could break through the denial: there would be this wonderful moment when Mr. Peterson would be in tears and I would be in tears and we would find ourselves at a deeper understanding of life and death.

Before entering his room, I could hear myself having these reactions and recognized that they would be damaging to the quality of the coming encounter.

I shifted my plan to listening to Mr. Peterson the best way I know how. To find out who he is. With this shift, I felt more grounded in my body (a sensation of how my weight is carried to the floor through my feet) and ready to see him.

Observations:

The room: This visit was made late morning. The weather during Mr. Peterson's stay had been consistently sunny and cool, but this day was overcast and gloomy and the room lights were off. There were two nurses working at the computer station when I entered the room and they soon left. His bed did not sit straight in the room as it had before but was turned slightly toward the window. As I had noted during previous visits, there were no indica-

tions that he had received any visitors during his stay: no cards, flowers, pictures, not much in the way of personal effects other than his glasses.

The chaplain: Entering the room I felt content, grounded, alert and with a refreshed sense of purpose as a chaplain following a meeting with the Spiritual Care Advisory Committee. I go and stand by the window side of his bed so that I'm not standing with my back to his nurses.

The patient: Mr. Peterson was semi-reclined in bed, with his feet exposed beneath the covers at the end of the bed. His feet were turned outwards awkwardly [no sense of feeling in his legs?] and had a discolored, scaly, and shiny appearance. I wondered if he has diabetic neuropathy.

Compared to my visit with him two days previously, his eyes were clouded and grey [like the sky]. His body seemed to be more sunk into the mattress than before, suggesting that his muscles were more relaxed, but also suggesting that he had less tone [life force]—that he was perhaps more resigned and less hopeful. His voice was still rich, deep and gravelly but there were more pauses. His voice was weaker, and he had less air behind each word.

Analysis – the Patient
Theological Concerns:

Mr. Peterson once had a faith of some degree, then lost it as his alcoholism took over, then rediscov-

ered it in the form of AA. His descriptions of this in earlier conversations were said clearly and without hesitation. Clearly, I should learn more about the role of God in AA—and I didn't take the best opportunity to start this learning by asking him to tell me more.

With that kind of background, I might have been able to better keep that God in the room with us during this conversation. For example, after hearing P7, who was this God he was addressing? What was he asking of this God? Looking at this now, I'm thinking he was asking to be taken not home but Home, meaning Heaven, that place of warmth and welcome and repose.

Psychological Concerns:
Denial—I don't have the clinical training to say if denial is present or not for Mr. Peterson. From a lay perspective, it is easy to say, "yes" because of his unwillingness to discuss the depth of his medical condition with any of his caregivers, but my untrained thought is that perhaps those things just didn't matter to him. What does he have to live for? He has survived a lifelong struggle with alcohol, something that he thinks robbed him of the chance of marriage and a family. He has no living family members.

More than all these things, I am deeply moved by his love of his home, one that he has lived in since *the age of 15. A home that his parents bought at a time before he became consumed by alcohol. In this visit and previous ones, I felt that his health was intimately entwined with the health of his home. He felt his home's symptoms — bad toilet, broken microwave — almost more than his own. He spoke of these things as if they were indeed symptoms to be addressed more than his own.*

So maybe he was in denial—he could have at least acknowledged the full depth of his medical condition and then said that it is not that import-ant to him. Granted, he didn't do that. But I'm left with a feeling of "so what?"

Maybe acceptance, as contrasted with denial, can be non-verbal. Maybe that is what happened between P6 and P7. The resignation that I noted in P7 was physical more than anything, a certain kind of relaxing and sinking of his body. Maybe that was his recognition of death's steady approach, and all he asked was to be taken home...

Sociological Concerns:

Here was a man who could easily be seen as someone alone. No family, his only friend an occasional care-taker who would come into his home to help him. [She was the one who was calling him during his hospitalization to talk house problems.]

Yet this was an insurance salesman. From his easy manner and his deep rich voice, I would guess a fairly successful salesman once he joined AA. His work was to help people like him, to help people trust him and he seemed to sustain those abilities at full strength.

Perhaps this life-long set of habits was part of the reason people thought he might be in denial or a "poor historian." He had an ability to focus on the needs and wishes of the person he was talking to rather than on his own. I don't remember any other patient I've encountered who would ask me, "How is your day going?" That question didn't feel like a deflection from his issues but a genuine question. Writing this now, I can almost imagine those being the last words he will ever say some day.

Ethical Concerns:
None come to mind. But having said that, I recognize that I really liked Mr. Peterson and that part of that "liking" was how much he seemed to like me.

Analysis — the Chaplain
I'll start with my reaction to hearing that a patient is a "poor historian." The reaction is anger that a patient should be labeled such a way. To me, after fifteen years of teaching about the therapeutic elements of the patient-physician relationship at the medical school in Hawaii, the label "poor historian" only applies to the physician who writes that

in the record. Such a physician is the poor historian and not the patient.

The patient's story, both verbal and non-verbal, is the patient's story. It is not the patient's job to order it into a neat and efficient form. It is not their job to answer all questions directly and to the point. It is the physician's job to create a useful story with the patient.

Ah, there is the arrogance and self-righteousness of me as a medical educator. "Here is how it is supposed to be done." But I'm not the doctor rushing from patient to patient, gathering the data I think necessary when determining treatment. I'm not the one charting on his patients at 8:00 at night, having missed dinner and his daughter's band concert. I don't really know how to take a medical history; I only know how to talk about it.

But I do know how to listen. That is my expertise. I feel that my job as chaplain is to do the work of hearing the history that perhaps few physicians can hear, and to contribute that to the progress notes. What wasn't said by the patient, but could have been? What was his body telling me, as compared to what his words were telling me?

Actually, my reaction to "denial" is not so different. Denial is not blocking access to useful information about the patient. Denial by itself is useful information. It is as much a part of the patient's history and story as anything else.

As for a critique of my performance, I can see several areas where I could have done better. At C3 I have essentially dismissed as unimportant the "symptoms" of his house. "No, don't talk about that. I want to talk about you." I think that represents my ego at play—"I'm going to find out things about you that no one else could find."

A more difficult question to answer is whether I ended the conversation too soon after hearing how tired he was. Did I see that as a chance to pull a polite exit, or did I sense that my work was done and nothing more was needed? I'd like to think I had a deep intuition that the shift from P6 to P7 was therapeutic and now I did best by stepping back and letting his sense of resignation soak in. But I can't say that for sure.

Let's come back to my sense of liking Mr. Peterson because he liked me. What do I do with patients who don't like me? Is there such a thing as a love (or "like") of any patient regardless of their reflection of those feelings? Or is that an abstract ideal? What do I give less of to patients that I don't like? Most likely, it is less intuition — I don't soak into them in the same way I felt with this patient.

Pastoral Opportunity

In my lineage of Zen, we place high value on seeing things truly or clearly. We acknowledge many forms of this ability. For example, there is the whole, the gestalt, and that includes not just the man inside his own skin but the man as part of a continuum with all that surrounds him, including his room, his caregivers, the weather, his story, his parents, and beyond.

Sometimes I have glimpses of such clarity, but then there is also the patient as he sees himself. How does that vision compare to a "true" vision? Yesterday, a friend told me, "Gordon, you get me," meaning that I saw/felt/perceived her as she saw herself. I think that form of seeing is what I most readily do with patients. I "get" them. Certainly, that has some therapeutic value to them—they have been witnessed. But the ongoing question for me is, "When I see them as they see themselves, when I see them through their own eyes, what else am I missing that might be valuable to their care?" No answer to this at the moment, but that is the opportunity this patient has opened for me.

End

This verbatim is a rookie's attempt—not much capture of dialogue, and several missed opportunities for deeper discussions with the patient. I would diagnose Mr. Peterson's spiritual problem as "a longing for a sense of home now that his home of fifty-three years may no longer be available," but I did little to address that problem other than acknowledging it. I also fell into a common trap of choosing a patient for a verbatim who makes me somehow look good, whether through a compliment paid or a key insight provided. This is less me learning than it is me wanting to look good.

This is the essence of the verbatim form. First, there is an effort to understand the context of the encounter. What do we already know of this patient? What is the state of mind of the chaplain before entering the room? What is the chaplain's plan? Then dialogue is captured, imperfectly, since there are no notes or recordings during the encounter, only a quick capture from memory once out of the patient's room. And then analysis after the fact, both of the patient and the chaplain. For the patient, we examine several dimensions: theological, psychological, sociological, and ethical. For the chaplain, the format is more free-form, a chance for self-reflection. And finally, discussion of "pastoral opportunity." What actually was the spiritual care needed in this encounter and how well was it was met?

What ink on paper cannot capture is the atmosphere once a verbatim is brought before one's CPE colleagues for discussion. In my program, written assignments were presented to the group by reading them aloud. As a reader, you see the words on a page but the group participants in the room with me were getting the feelings that lay behind my words.

For example, I was unconscious of the fact, when I met Mr. Peterson and when I was writing this verbatim, that he reminded me of the father of my first girlfriend: the same deep voice, the same sincere question of "How are you?" There was something similar about his hair and the shape of his head, his work as an insurance salesman. Mr. Youtzy was a man that I loved in some fashion, and that love mixed in with the love I had for his daughter. So, my awkward question about love at the end of my own analysis is just the tip of the iceberg of what I was feeling in that room, talking with my colleagues.

How do I know? Because at the end of the discussion of my verbatim, Scott said, "I wish I could be your patient. Then I might know the kind of love you provided him." I was taken aback, not knowing how to answer. So, I didn't. Was that a compliment or a complaint?

One lesson I learned during these three months was that we cannot freely use emotions, memories, ideas, that we are unconscious of. In this sense, the goal of CPE training was to bring as much of ourselves as possible into awareness so that the tools we have available for any given encounter are that much more abundant.

5.
He has resolved the question of life and death.

The writing assignments during CPE never seemed to end. Immediately following the first verbatim, the next piece of writing was something called a "theological reflection paper." In this assignment, we were asked to look at ourselves in the mirror of a particular piece of liturgy.

The text assigned to me was the story often known as "The Four Signs," about the transformation of the historical figure Siddhartha into the religious figure of the Buddha. For those unfamiliar, it's a story akin to how Jesus became Christ. In our writing, we were asked to be guided by questions such as "How do you see yourself in this passage?" or "How is this passage a metaphor for what you are experiencing?" Although this is a key story in Buddhism, there is no one orthodox text.

The Four Signs

The primordial story of how Buddhism came into being begins in 560 BC, the year when a son was born to King Suddhodana, ruler of the Shakya clan in northern India, and his wife Mahamaya. This baby was given the name Siddhartha, and it was prophesized that he would become a great king if he remained as part of his father's household or would become the Supremely Enlightened One if he did not.

King Suddhodana deeply wanted his son to become a great ruler, and thus he did everything he could to make Siddhartha's life as comfortable and meaningful as possible, all the while training him as he grew in all the arts required of a leader. And when the time came, he presented him with a bride: the beautiful and regal Yashodhara.

Despite the comfort and ease of his life within the palace, there came a time when Siddhartha asked to see more of the world outside the palace walls. Wanting to please his son, the King asked Siddhartha's servant Channa to arrange an outing to a nearby market. On the appointed day, Channa and Siddhartha set out from the East Gate of his father's palace.

Channa had done as the King had requested. The market was vibrant, clean and full of youth and energy. Siddhartha was enjoying all the sights, but what most caught his attention was a man walking slowly with a staff in his hand, stooped over, his face deeply furrowed in the way a field looks after plowing, and a long white beard.

"Who is this?" Siddhartha asked.

And Channa answered, "This is an old man."

"What's wrong with him?"

"Nothing. That is what happens to us all as the years pass."

Siddhartha returned home, bothered by this image of aging. His father, noticing his distraction, sought to make Siddhartha's palace life even more luxurious.

Some time went by before Siddhartha asked Channa to get ready for another excursion outside the palace walls. This time they left by the north gate, going further into the town. Channa had prepared for this trip well. The town was clean and the people appeared happy. But as they turned a corner, Siddhartha glimpsed a man whose eyes were wild with a high fever. His body was wracked by a cough.

"What's wrong with him?" Siddhartha asked.

And Channa answered, "That is a sick man, someone whose body is ill. Someday, in some fashion, this happens to us all."

Siddhartha returned home, bothered by his memory of the sick man. His father, noticing his distraction, sought to make Siddhartha's palace life even more luxurious.

More time passed, and Siddhartha asked for another outing. On this one, despite Channa's efforts to make sure only pleasant sights would be encountered, they came across a procession of people weeping. At the front was a man on a litter, looking as if he might be sleeping, his arms crossed over his chest.

"Why is that man sleeping?" asked Siddhartha.

And Channa answered, "He is not sleeping; he is

dead. This is the fate that awaits us all."

Hearing this, Siddhartha was bothered even more than before. If all people age, get sick and then die, what is the purpose of living? He returned home, deeply troubled.

Siddhartha waited a long time before he asked Channa to go out into the town one more time. By now, Channa realized there was no point trying to hide the reality of life from Siddhartha. Without any preparations, they headed out of the west gate, headed to a market in a neighboring town. As they arrived at the edge of the market, Siddhartha saw a man, neither young nor old, with a shaven head. This man was walking along in a clean but plain robe, an eating bowl hanging from his sash, chanting in a deep voice as he walked.

"What is this?" Siddhartha asked.

"This is a holy man," Channa answered.

"Why does he look so serene in the midst of the turmoil of this market?"

"Because he has resolved the question of life and death."

This was the moment Siddhartha had been waiting for. He had found a way out of the despair he felt knowing that all humans age, all humans get sick, and all humans die.

It was not an easy choice, but one night not long after, Siddhartha took one last look at his sleeping wife and his new baby, and he set off toward the mountains with a conviction that he too must resolve the question of life and death. His father would be saddened, but Siddhartha felt that he had fulfilled some part of his obligation to his family by leaving behind a child. He knew that he could never return.

The life he lived from this point, the austerities he faced, the training he embraced are all part of another story. But the night he left the palace was the birth of Buddhism. Siddhartha was able to fulfill the prophecy that he would become the Supremely Enlightened One. And his four experiences — old age, sickness, death, and the recognition of a human able to convey fearlessness without words — became what is known as the Four Signs.

Now, how can I claim this story as part of my story? I've never asked this of myself so it's a bit awkward. I, too, came from a life of ease and comfort. My parents and my sisters loved me. Our life was not luxurious, but it was comfortable. I was smart enough and loved learning, so school was a wonderful challenge and I found excellent teachers who could feed and enlarge that love.

I had grandparents who grew old, who suffered illness and who died, but those experiences seemed on the periphery of my life. Of course my grandparents were important to me, of course their deaths were inevitable, but they didn't disturb my fundamental sense that the universe was a place with more joys than sorrows, that my curiosity would always be fed, and that there was an order to the universe best expressed through the languages of mathematics and physics.

Looking back, I see how that belief in the powers of mathematics and physics was a shield for me, a way to protect myself from a deep sense of inadequacy — "I will never be good enough, strong enough, to understand everything I want to understand, not good enough to do everything I want to do." That sensation was there before my first marriage ended in divorce, but the divorce took it in a whole new direction and to a whole new depth. My experience of divorce proved how weak mathematics and logic and physics were, weak because they could not help me understand why my wife divorced me.

This experience was the crack in the shell of my self-constructed universe. The forces of the universe were far stronger than any I had imagined possible. The scale of the universe went far beyond any boundaries I could imagine.

In the years after the divorce—training intensely in Zen, living with very little money, aching to be able to live with my two children—I found myself identifying most strongly with people whose lives were a mess. Maybe they were estranged from family, maybe they had no money, maybe they had no friends, but I was so impressed that they could still be alive in the face of all this adversity.

I remember a conversation with a woman who had come for several weeks of Zen training. She was offended that I was not vegetarian, as she was. "How can you call yourself a Buddhist and still justify eating meat?" Kate wanted to know.

I in turn was offended by her sense of self-righteousness and told her that few people in the world had a lot of choices they could make about their diets. The majority of humans ate what they had to, and not what they wanted to. I found myself saying to Kate, "Who am I that I get to eat better than anyone else? Who am I to say that this food is better for me than that food? I could never live with myself that way."

I remember feeling surprised hearing these words come out of my mouth, but they felt true. Whatever the human experience, I felt that I had no fundamental right to say that is not my experience. That I get to choose what of human experience is OK for me to experience and what part is not OK for me to experience. To say "not OK" just seemed wrong—not in a moral sense but in a way that seemed to violate the nature of the universe.

Looking back, I sense that I may have always had this craving: to feel all of human experience deep in my bones and to not flinch, not judge, not complain as I feel it. My childhood form of this was an intense desire to know how the physical world worked, but my adult form was an intense desire to feel all the forces that drive human behavior. Previous to writing this reflection, my expression of this desire was to say that I wanted to "understand human behavior," but that is still the intellectual expression. The gut level is this discovery that I want to "feel human behavior."

It was only once I was in graduate school, at age 28, that I found my own holy man. This was Tenshin Tanouye Roshi. Like the holy man seen during Siddhartha's fourth excursion from his palace, he had resolved the question of life and death. I knew that I wanted that too.

I trained with him initially as a beginner—with hesitation, doubt, and a profound sense of inadequacy. But with my divorce at age 33, there became an urgency to push myself past my limits. I felt so close to death emotionally that any other form of life or training that might seem deadly had lost its power to scare me.

I entered Zen as a way to end my suffering. That was the promise of the Four Noble Truths, the first of the Buddha's teachings after his enlightenment experience. The goal of training is to end attachments because those are the source of suffering. Not easy, but at least clear. And this may be the most common perception of Buddhism in this country; Buddhists don't suffer because they have learned to take away attachments.

There is no polite way to respond to that statement other than to say, "Show me the person who doesn't have attachments." I haven't met such a person. Instead, I met a teacher who wasn't attached to his attachments, who could see through his attachments such that they didn't have the power to lock him in an endless cycle of suffering. And his method was Zen and swordsmanship.

But here too was language to be wary of. As you practice swinging a sword hour after hour, you can be fooled by the instruction to "cut your attachments." It isn't the attachments that are cut. It is the You that is cut. If attachments have no place to attach to, what power do they have?

The common language of "take away attachments" causes endless problems because it leaves the You intact, trying to scrape off those bloodsucking attachments. In this case, the attachments are not the problem, the You is the problem. Resolve the nature of You, and attachments have no more power. This was training I wanted. I wanted that attachment to my children. I didn't want that taken away. I just didn't want to suffer so much from it.

This gets at my compulsion to learn how to face suffering. I wasn't asking for my suffering to end. Out of some deep instinct, I knew I wanted to face it.

My first marriage ended painfully, with our children aged two and five at the time. I moved into a house two miles away from their mother, and for one year we shared custody. I continued in my work as a research scientist. Although that experience of shared custody was painful, I didn't steal away to my Zen teacher's dojo in the night. Instead, I carefully planned all the steps of my move over many months, including consultation with a child psychologist about ways to mitigate the impact of my move on my children.

But I didn't ask my children's opinion about the move, knowing their obvious answer. And I still left.

6.
Cassandra and Alexander the Great.

The physical and emotional intensity of CPE training kept building and, after a month of training, this week felt like the toughest one to date, primarily because it was forcing me to look at my marriage in ways that I wanted to avoid. I felt exhausted, inadequate, and sad. But also fully engaged.

On some level, I knew that this was what I had signed up for. I felt increasingly exposed, naked in front of patients, naked in front of my CPE colleagues, naked in front of myself. I wasn't sure what it was, but I wanted something inside me to change. And I was too committed in this search to back down.

It was a married couple that brought things to a head. Alex was a middle-age man, married to Cass for nine years. He was the patient, admitted to the hospital with abdominal pain.

Additional Factual Information:

When I first saw Alex during my 24-hour weekend call, he was awake and his wife Cass was present. Their story of their life together seemed to overwhelm the story of Alex's immediate illness, serious as it was. Both of them had previously diagnosed psychiatric problems. No money for rent [though he works as a bartender/waiter] and they are about to be kicked out of their apartment, no money for heat, no friends, no insurance.

Cass saw no hope for their future. Alex disagreed, "It always works out." But this triggered louder lamenting from her that he was a dreamer and couldn't see the truth.

After my initial visit with Alex, I spoke with his nurse, asking what is done when a spouse stays full-time in the hospital not out of concern for the patient, but because they have nowhere else to go. I was worried the Cass might be interfering with Alex's care.

The nurse seemed eager to vent and took me into a side room. "We are seeing more and more homelessness. It wasn't like this before. It is hard on all of us. She is way more demanding than he is, and he is the one who is sick." I asked if there was anyplace else Cass could go in the hospital so he could get some peace. The nurse said, "Not really. I don't want her sleeping in the family lounge." I left the first encounter with the patient and his wife feeling helpless to attend to their needs.

Plans:

Having read Alex's chart [notes from the physician, social worker, and morning nurses] before going in for this second visit, I asked his nurse how he was doing. My goal was to provide the patient with some sense of strength, readying him for his return to a difficult life. The nurse said that they had been getting ready to discharge Alex today, but that now they were worried about heart symptoms and were running more tests.

I asked whether his wife was still agitated. The nurse said that she was not in the room and was most likely in the family lounge. I thought, "Good! Finally, I'll get some time just with him." With his wife present, I felt that Alex could not speak easily about his own fears or concerns, and I wanted to explore these with him.

Observations:

Given my earlier encounters with the seeming help-lessness of this patient's living condition, this was not an easy room to step into. Cass was unexpected-ly present, sitting on the couch amidst tangled sheets and clothes, wearing a hospital gown. The shades

*were drawn almost shut. The room smelled of hu-
man sweat, smelling stronger as I got closer to the
wife. Unlike previous visit, Alex was not antic. His
smile was less forced—still friendly and genuine, but
less of a mask. Still, his angry wife was the strongest
source of gravity in the room.*

The visit: (C: Chaplain, P: Patient, W: Wife)

C1: *Hi there. It's been awhile since I stopped by.
I heard you might be leaving today so I wanted to come by and see how you are doing. [I'm
standing on the hall side of the patient's bed at
this point.]*

P1: *Nope. Not yet. More tests today. I passed out
in the bathroom.*

C2: *Is that good news or bad news? [moving to the
foot of the bed in order to stand closer to Cass]*

P2: *Hey! [talking to his wife] Move that stuff off
the chair so the chaplain can sit. [I help her
bundle up clothes, which she moves beside her
on the couch. The chair is right beside his wife,
close to the corner of his bed. The movement of
the clothes stirs the air and the smell of stale
human sweat in the room gets even stronger.
I sit down and lean back like I'm there for a
relaxed conversation with friends.]*

C3: *So, what's happening?*

W1: *I'm going to kill somebody [said with her familiar anger. Alex grimaces as she says this.]*

C4: That bad, hunh?

W2: Dude! The fucking computer doesn't work. *[She must have been down in the family lounge in order to use the internet...]* And I'm still the invisible one. No one wants to see me, hear me. Nobody wants to smell me. They didn't want me to have this gown but I'm sorry, I can't keep stinking up clothes. All I've got is this sweat-shirt and if I keep wearing it while I go up and down stairs *[here at the hospital—but, why no elevator...?]*, it will stink. I've got nothing else to wear... *[I'm looking at Cass at first, but then I glance over at Alex to see how he is taking this all in. He looks powerless.]*

C5: Well, I can see you *[talking to Cass]*. I can hear you. I had to stay over in the hospital Sunday night, and I didn't take a shower before working yesterday. I didn't like smelling myself either. This place is supposed to be so clean and tidy. No stink allowed...

W3: Yeah, no poor people allowed...But that's their problem. We still have no place to go.

C6: I hear you...so, *[I turn to Alex]* what happened to you last night? *[He looks eager to answer now that the attention has come back to him.]*

P3: Whoa! I got so dizzy *[said happily, like he's glad to have a real symptom]*. I got up to take a piss and I was filling the whole bottle. I mean, I was filling that whole thing up — it *was just pouring out of me. And maybe it was just too much because I suddenly got dizzy. And I'm looking for a place to set it before I go down...*

C7: *And then you fainted?*

P4: *Yeah, straight down.*

C8: *Wow! I'm glad you didn't hit your head.*

W4: *Dude! That would have been a mess if you had dropped it. God, the smell would have killed me.*

C9: *And then what?*

P5: *Well, the doctor heard about it this morning and he's wondering about my heart now, so they want to run tests before I can go.*

C10: *I wasn't kidding about the good news/bad news thing. What do you think? You've been on a roller coaster with this discharge/no discharge thing. Are you OK being here a bit longer?*

W5: *Why doesn't anybody ask me that question? He's getting all the drugs. He's getting all the tests. I can't get nothing. I'm the bad guy. Always I'm the bitch. People look right through me.*

C11: *But you [said to Cass] understand that most people here see your husband as their patient, right? I've never seen a double bed here where they can plop you both in the same bed—you guys would need the deluxe version where each half of the bed has its own mechanics—yours can go up, but his can go down. I can't see you guys agreeing on how to arrange the pillows.*

P6:*[Laughs] You got that right! We can leave her right over there on the couch!*

C12: *Those drugs might help you, you know... [referring to the bi-polar medications she supposedly left in the place where they were staying] Can anybody give you a ride to get your meds?*

W6: *Dude! I already told you about that bus transfer place. You think I want more of that "Hey, Baby...How about it?" crap? And do you think we've got friends? He called his boss last night, asking about the money from that employee fund. All that guy had to say was "When are you coming back to work?" No "How are you doing?" Nothing!*

C13: *[Talking to the patient] Maybe you should do some of that pissing in the bottle at work. You know, you might just get dizzy again and who knows if you could keep from dropping it on the floor a second time. Whoops – sorry.*

P7: *[Laughs] Yeah! That would be just about right for him [the boss].*

...several more minutes of talk about their life once they get out of the hospital. Talking more about looking for work, trying to find a local library with internet access, Cass's body odor etc....then, in closing:

C14: *So, what do you think? [talking to Alex] If you could become anybody, who would you be?*

W7: Cassandra! I don't have to become her—I am her. The gods cursed me to always speak the truth but have no one believe me.

P8: Yeah, and I've thought about being Alexander the Great.

C15: Yes indeed, I look at that profile and you look like you belong on a coin. [His wife does a belly laugh.] You know, Halloween is coming up and I think I can see you both pulling this off— Cassandra and Alexander [more laughter] ...I do need to get going to see more patients now, but I'm going to keep thinking of you both. You guys have got guts. Don't give up!

W8: No way, dude!

P9: I haven't seen anybody make Cass laugh like this. I'm going to keep thinking of you.

Analysis — the Patient
Theological Concerns:

Over the course of my CPE work to date, I've been asking myself how I best serve patients in my role as a chaplain. I've come through a phase of recognizing how valuable it can be for patients to feel seen, gotten, heard, accepted. From the perspective of the training of a Zen priest, that is indeed the primary work: "to become one with" is the phrase used. That is not a "become one with" in your imagination, but in a deeply visceral sense.

The reason we stop there in describing the

work—I think—is that once there has been that joining, whatever happens next emerges from a different context than the one in which there is a concrete patient here and a concrete chaplain over there.

But over the course of the last few weeks, I haven't been satisfied that "becoming one with" and then allowing the "more" to just emerge is sufficient. The pump has to be primed in order for the "more" to flow correctly. To this end, Pruyser offers a useful challenge with his seven diagnostic domains. The challenge I feel is that it is not enough to simply see a patient through their own eyes. Instead, when I can see through those eyes, how can I (meaning we) alter the nature of the reality we are experiencing?

In other words, if I perceive that a patient suffers from an inability to experience the Holy in their life, can I (we) work from within to facilitate movement towards that experience? It becomes an unconscious intention in other words and what I now realize that such an intention may not work intentionally unless the seed already exists in me as a chaplain.

Those things we see as diagnostic may also become therapeutic. Diagnosing an inability to experience the Holy also suggests the work to be done: namely, facilitating a patient's search for the Holy. I say "suggests" carefully because the facilitation I am describing can never effectively be done from outside the patient's own experience. I feel that it can only be done from within that sensation of "becoming one with."

I'm choking on my own words here a bit as I explore this expanded notion of chaplaincy for myself. I am writing with scarcely any experience of actually encountering a patient in this expanded fashion. But I am struck by the lives of Alex and Cass. It would be easy to say that their basic needs for food, clothing, shelter and health are so far from being met that it makes no sense to think of their needs for spiritual care.

Let's first go for healthcare and rent support so that they can live in a less dangerous neighborhood, and closer to food banks. Then, once we've handled that, they become worthy of a chaplain's help in exploring the Divine. I trust my readers recognize my sarcastic tone, but it is one directed at myself. Their need for the Divine is now, not later. What can I (we) do about that from the perspective of "becoming one with?" I don't know.

Psychological Concerns

There are so many directions we could go when considering Alex's psychological concerns but the one that first comes to mind: Why this particular dynamic between the patient and his wife? It clearly is a well-honed coping mechanism: Cass is the angry bitch and he is the happy-go-lucky guy, friend to all of mankind.

Given his wife's harsh and bitter persona, this is not a couple likely to have much success navigating life in normal society. And this is a man not likely to be able to focus attention on his own needs. Cass will never generate in others a desire to help her unless there is someone ready to walk into her particular version of Hell. Alex will never be able to seek the kind of medical help he so obviously needs until he takes control of his needs instead of allowing her to dictate them.

Several questions come to mind. How did they hit upon this coping mechanism? Did they ever have a chance for another coping mechanism? How well does this one serve them? Are they stuck with it?

At first glance, my label for this couple is "train wreck" or "dysfunctional family." But "dysfunctional" is a tricky term. My feeling is that until anyone could explore the way in which their roles actually serve a useful purpose, there is no way any shift could take place.

Out of the various professions who might encounter this couple—chaplain, social worker, physician, psychologist—I actually think a chaplain might have the most useful attitude and framework with which one could approach them. There is just about everything to "fix" for Alex and Cass, but my feeling is that this is one of those existential situations where the best approach is to recognize that not only is there no way to "fix" things for them, but to recognize first that there is nothing that needs "fixing." That may sound bizarre, but until one first finds and accepts their current, not potential, humanity, nothing more can happen.

Ethical Concerns
I felt comfortable joining into their lives but did not feel a need for any kind of aggressive advocacy role with regards to his care. The medical care he was given seemed no different than the care provided to any other patient.

I am concerned, though, that I focused more on Cass than on the patient himself. There were at least three sets of problems in their room: the problems the patient has, the problems his wife has, and the problems that exist in the two of them together. I felt that the bulk of my work focused on the last problem, and some of the work focused just on her, but that didn't leave much attention for the patient himself and that doesn't feel right.

Analysis — the Chaplain
This is the hardest section of this verbatim to write because it hits close to home for me. Initially, I felt very much engaged with Alex because his life and his dilemma presented such a clear cry for help. There are no easy answers to his medical problems; there are even fewer answers to his social, emotional, spiritual problems.

This is a true example of a situation where the only possible approach lies in "being" and not "doing," at least from a chaplaincy perspective. I often feel most engaged in these situations. So that was what brought me back to this patient for a second visit, even though he wasn't on any of my assigned units and I had no formal responsibility for providing his spiritual care.

But Cass plays such a large role in the issues raised by his hospitalization and I have come to recognize in the course of developing this verbatim—especially as I was recreating the conversation in the room —that I have a lot of self-identification with this patient. This is painful to admit, but worth exploring. Just like good theatre takes human behavior and exaggerates it to a point beyond reality, I find the extreme coping mechanisms this patient and his wife display point a finger straight to my own heart.

My wife came through a stretch of time in which she could suddenly erupt in anger, verbally so, to myself, but more painfully, she did this with other people important to me. In the face of this, my role was to be the peacemaker, the Zen guy above it all, the guy who could explain why my wife would erupt and ask for understanding from those she hurt. This was the coping mechanism we were locked into and it took a long time for me to see how damaging it was—to her, to me, to all around us.

How false that coping mechanism was. Part of

the coping was that I so clearly thought of the anger as her problem; I was just another one of the victims but because of my Zen training, I could rise above it. This was the story I told myself.

But once I got in touch with my own anger about my marriage, things began to shift. I had to do two things: abandon that coping mechanism and be willing to risk the chaos that ensued; and I had to recognize how intimately I was tied into my wife's anger. I wasn't separate from it. I was part of it. I had to acknowledge that I was causing her anger.

I feel embarrassed to admit such things. Having already gone through a divorce, having lived to age 61, having trained for 40 years in Zen, you would think I could do better than this, and not allow my life to hurt others.

Up until now, I had hidden the struggles of my marriage from my parents. But I asked my mother for help a few weeks ago. I laid out my pain and she heard it. She shared times of pain in her own life, in her own marriage. She had no intention to fix anything but was able to join me in a new state of just living and not coping. And she helped me open up to you [my CPE colleagues]...I share this with you so you can help me remain raw and open to life, and to patients.

My ability to sit easily besides this patient's raging wife, unpleasant in so many ways, has been hard-earned. The healing I sought to bring Cass and Alex is some of what I have only begun to expe-

rience for myself. By living out their pain so clearly and helping me to better see mine, Alex and Cass gave me healing as well.

Pastoral Opportunity

The opportunity is to not lie. Don't pretend all is well. Say how painful this is. Don't look for a new coping mechanism—live with the rawness.

I've been acknowledged for my strengths for so many years—basically since becoming a medical educator 20 years ago and receiving my designation as a Zen master from my teacher then—that I have swept far under the rug many years of helplessness I experienced earlier my life. I thought I had earned the right to say that I succeeded, that I overcame so many emotional barriers, that I no longer had to look back.

But when I do look back, I see myself looking at myself today. There are many strengths in my life now but there are also moments of fresh helplessness. I need to recognize those for the sake of my patients.

End

One month into my chaplaincy training, it had become quite raw. I started this verbatim by expressing a sense of helplessness and ended it the same way. Finally, I'm letting my supervisor Jeff and, more importantly, letting Scott, Collin and Linda hear my vulnerability. The tough guy act was gone, my persona as a former medical school faculty member was gone. This became a turning point in my relationship with them.

But it was a strange kind of helplessness, because I also felt quite at ease with Alex and his wife. They stirred strong emotions, which helped me understand this sense of ease with them. Still, I did not feel that this was competent chaplaincy work for a number of reasons. Primarily, I was too focused on Cass and did little to explore Alex's needs for care. Notice, for example, his ready identification with Alexander the Great. That would have been a perfect opportunity to ask him to tell me more about himself as Alexander.

There is also this sense that there is nothing that needs "fixing." Clearly, I was resisting the labels that might ordinarily be placed on this couple. Instead, I was asking for an understanding of the "logic" of their coping mechanisms. There is a chance that I am protecting them in the same manner that I was protecting myself in my own marriage.

This brings me to a larger point about the nature of chaplaincy training. The basic effort is to craft a "therapeutic self," meaning that the chaplain becomes the instrument of healing. For that to work, as in other healing professions like clinical psychology, there must be transparency. By this, I mean that a chaplain does well to be aware of the emotions that patient work brings up. If those emotions remain unconscious, they most likely will play out in self-serving ways.

As with Alex and Cass, I may have been seeking unconsciously to heal myself more than I was healing them. If the emotions are conscious, however, a chaplain has more freedom in their actions. There is a "seeing through" the emotions, a recognition that something has been triggered in one's self. That gives us the freedom to notice it and set it aside, before continuing with work that's appropriate.

At this point in our CPE training, we had just been introduced to a way of viewing the role of anxiety in people's lives, our own included. Before starting CPE, I had felt that anxiety was a relatively minor emotion, not often a part of my life. I struggled with the perspective that anxiety was the predominant forcefield of our emotional lives, present to a greater or lesser extent in everyone at all times. Those people who avoid getting snarled in the anxiety forcefield, either their own or that of other people, are said to be "self-differentiated."

Becoming more and more free of anxiety is one of the most prominent goals of chaplaincy training. I was a long way from this goal. But I can report that Patricia and I healed our relationship. The key step for me was letting go of my stance that I was above all of the turmoil between us. Instead, I had to plunge into the turmoil, allowing the distinction between her issues and my issues to soften. Confronting the painful relationship between Cassandra and Alexander the Great had been the first step.

7.
Defeated, decisively, by constantly greater beings.

The next week, all the emotions building during the previous weeks finally came to a boil. My risk-taking went too far, leading to a confrontation with a colleague and my letter of resignation.

The risk-taking was with a patient, an encounter that I turned into a verbatim for presentation. I had started out, pleased with myself as I pulled together the familiar elements, pleased with what I thought I learned. But that was before I presented this verbatim to Jeff and my CPE colleagues. What would have ordinarily been a one-hour discussion became a three-hour whirlwind.

Lee was a middle-aged man with a freshly-received diagnosis of cancer. I went in to his room with two clear goals: to take comfort with someone who might be feeling as miserable as I was, and to see how I might work with a patient who had repeatedly turned down the offer of a visit by other chaplains on the team.

In hindsight, I would have been wise to speak with my supervisor before proceeding with such a visit, but I didn't. I had been learning hard and fast for five weeks and felt more than ready to push my boundaries.

The goal of seeing a patient who had rejected chaplain visits may seem odd; it was a violation of a chaplain's usual protocol. But recall my interest in the concept of minister as spiritual care clinician, one who both diagnoses and treats.

I knew that the medical staff would be appropriate in working with a patient who was refusing nursing care or a physician's care. The patient might resist but almost always the staff would find a way to provide the necessary care. I didn't accept that spiritual care would be viewed any differently. If there was reason to believe that it might be of value for the patient's well-being, why would care be withheld? Good logical reasoning there, easy to justify in my own mind, given many years of experience working with medical residents in hospitals.

At this point, I still felt a greater affinity with medical residents in their care for patients than I did with my fellow chaplains. I wasn't interested in a type of chaplaincy that was simply caring and comforting. I wanted a type that gave a patient courage, that gave them a new view of themselves and their healing, that got them out of the hospital sooner than what might be the normal course of their stay.

My ideal was a muscular chaplaincy, a deeply insightful chaplaincy, a courageous chaplaincy. This was my frame of mind on this Monday. My need to become this kind of chaplain was more important than patient needs, than the needs of my colleagues.

The patient who became part of my risk-taking had been admitted a few days before with a preliminary diagnosis of "abdominal pain with evidence of a 3.5 cm left renal mass...Epigastric pain with mild symptoms suggestive of reflux and stomach wall thickening."

Additional Factual Information:

Lee came to the emergency room two days before I met with him. He had been released from prison two weeks prior to admission. Following his release, he had enjoyed a week of good health, but then began feeling abdominal pains and symptoms he had not experienced before. Following a CT scan done after coming to the ER, the patient was told that he has "what appears to be a renal cell carcinoma." You and I would say "kidney cancer."

Plans:

My plan for the day was to see as many patients as possible who had said "no" to a chaplain visit.

For a warmup, I visited two men who had already shown various degrees of resistance to a chap-

lain visit. With the first patient, I made no head-way. There was five minutes of dialogue, but no dents in his certainty that he had no spiritual issues.

The second patient I saw was one I'd seen the day before, a man admitted for alcohol detoxifica-tion and whose wife had just announced that they were divorcing. On the first visit, we exchanged a few pleasantries, and he then dismissed me, saying "Well, thanks for coming by."

On today's visit, I got a bit inside his defenses. When he dismissed me again early in the conver-sation: "OK. That's enough for now." I just kept talking as if I didn't hear him and we were able over the next fifteen minutes to get to some substance in discussion of his suffering before he hit his limit. [his new limit—he was stretched by the encounter and so was I.]

But for this third patient of the day, the odds of success looked slim. Lee had come in for abdominal pain and found out that it was kidney cancer. Ac-cording to his nurses, he wasn't accepting the diag-nosis as real. He told them, "It makes no sense." Lee had an intimidating manner, reinforced by seeing the note in his chart of his recent prison term. One CPE chaplain intern had visited him this morning and was turned away. I had chosen him for a visit because he fit the theme of the day.

Before this, I had always respected the ex-pression of a decline of a chaplain visit, no matter *how presented. I thought this was the profession-al thing to do. But I often wondered why I should back off so easily when a physician or a nurse would rarely do so. The patient is here for treatment so how is a chaplain different from a nurse or a doctor with regards to a patient's care? I've seen nurses and doctors be respectful and stra-tegically insistent when a patient declined their help. I wanted to see what I could learn about this attitude for myself.*

With Lee, I felt like I had little to lose. My strategy would be to somehow humble myself and ask for his help in learning how to provide pastoral care to someone who doesn't want it. I felt stupid and unconfident walking in with such a plan, but at least I would have an excuse if I got rejected. By calling this an experiment, I was more prepared for failure than if I went in there with my usual, self-confident, chaplain persona.

We had an awkward start—I'm surprised we got through it—but once we found our rhythm, Lee was off and running, speaking very fast, sometimes with an accent that was unintelligible. His speaking style seemed to come from his time in prison. I've learned over the years how inmates learn to speak one-on-one in a crowded room. That speech is rap-id, often coded, and pitched in a way to just catch the listener's ear while the speaker never loses an awareness of the surroundings.

Observations:

Lee was lying in bed, very alert, when I walked in. He was on the phone but ended the conversation. The room was dark because the shades were drawn. There were no personal effects. His tray table had an unusually neat assembly of the usual tissues, water jug, lunch menu. His eyes were very strong and clear and challenging—I felt seen in a glance. His alertness was visceral, his muscle tone felt like he could leap out of bed in a second. He didn't seem ill at all.

The visit:

C1: *I'm Gordon, one of the chaplains here. I've got some questions for you.*

P1: *Like what?*

C2: *I know you saw a chaplain earlier today and you turned her down. I'm here to learn how to be a chaplain and I want to learn how to talk with someone even when they don't want to talk. I know you did some time locked up [in prison — his eyes go empty at this statement — a very eerie sensation to see happen] so I figure you don't put up with any kind of bullshit from a preacher...*

P2: *Don't you go cursing in here... [said with little apparent emotion]*

C3: *I'm sorry. I'm not a Christian. I'm a Buddhist priest. [What kind of excuse is that!? I feel like I am really fumbling...] I've got nothing to sell you, but I do want to learn. Will you help me?*

P3: *Who told you to come in here? That doctor? Listen, you don't know anything about me. Why do you put that prison thing on me? I'm just like anybody else—inside, outside...I'm not any different with a man from how I am with a woman. No different with a doctor or a thief. You're coming at me like you just pulled one card out of a deck: the prison card. Man, that's just dumb. There are 51 other cards. You've got to play the whole deck. Otherwise, I'll get you with my mind game every time [he points a strong finger straight to the side of his head—that does feel menacing...]*

See, I can tell you I've got a nice car for sale outside. All you've got to do is get $25,000 cash and it's yours. So, you go get the $25,000 and bring it back. See—you ain't never seen the car. You've never seen if there even is a car, and you are standing there with $25,000 in your pocket. I got you. That money is mine. See—I got you smiling now. I got inside your head. You played one card and I played the whole deck. You've got to be way smarter than that—your face should never change. Don't let them read you.

By this point, Lee is off and running. Talking extremely fast, using his eyes to occasionally lock onto mine, gesturing with that same forefinger. This is one healthy looking and acting guy.

The subject matter ranges far and wide, including how to flirt, how to handle an angry wife, how to take care of your mother, how to raise your kids, how to work a job, how to handle other inmates in jail, how to manage several girlfriends at once, why he loved his grandmother ["She taught me everything. I could have been a preacher because of her."] As hard as it was to follow everything Lee said, it was strong and coherent. This man could have been a preacher...Here are some other excerpts from the long conversation:

> **P4**: *You think they can scare me? Scare me? I got this sheet [a 1-page information sheet about kidney cancer sitting on his bed-side table] telling me I've got cancer and you think anything can scare me? I'm a dead man but I've still got some living to do. [This is not a man in denial. Lee described how he hates pity and he is going to live this one out his way...] I got the money. I got the time...I hate to fly but I'm getting on a boat and going to Hawaii. I'm going to sit back and just do nothing. You know what I mean?*
> **C4**: *Yes. I lived there. I can smell that air.*

> *... more lessons from him...*

> **C5**: *You taught me today, thanks.*
> **P5**: *No, you taught me. You taught me by coming in humble. I know you went to college. I know*

you know lots of words. But I'm the one who survives, any place, any time. You respected that.

C6: *Well, really I came to work today feeling like shit because my wife and I had an argument yesterday. [Another long interlude about women who want to argue...] When I came in to the hospital today, I was feeling so bad, I figured if there was anybody here who might be feeling that kind of bad, it would be you. So, I wanted to come see you, and not get turned away....*

Funny thing—you tell your Mom that I think you are the healthiest guy in the hospital [because of his strong spirit].

P6: *Yeah, that's what my doctor told me.*

C7: *I want to come back tomorrow. Is that OK?*

P7: *I don't know...I may be gone. But I could teach you to preach!*

C8: *Yeah, I'd like that. I could be a Buddhist preacher.*

P8: *OK, but you're going to have to pay me for the lessons. [We both laugh.] See, I got you [meaning that I was surprised Lee would expect to be paid for his lessons. I didn't see that coming— he got me again.]*

Analysis — the Patient

A key theme of this long conversation was "mind games"—how to use them to your advantage and how to avoid them when directed at yourself. Lee's metaphor for these games was how many cards are being played from a deck of cards at any given time.

It is beyond the scope of this verbatim to explore why Lee might have felt this was the best way to talk with me. His long "lessons" felt more like streams of consciousness than strategic instruction. And, there may have been as much as one-third of his words that never registered with me. Now that I think of it, I listened to him as I am forced to do with someone speaking Japanese. I can catch some of the vocabulary as it streams by, but the "work" of listening is to watch for tone, atmosphere, body language and to derive meaning from those more than the words chosen.

The meaning I felt in Lee out of the avalanche of words was "I will survive." That's different from "I will live." It meant he will continue to live on his own terms. He has a well-constructed and well-articulated moral code with regards to his conduct and his relationships with others. The feeling was that he will stay true to his code until he dies. Don't give an inch!

Analysis — the Chaplain
Here's my main focus in writing this verbatim: I deliberately used this patient and I've got to figure out what that means. I used the two patients I saw before him. I came into the hospital this Monday morning feeling miserable, an unusual sensation for me during this CPE experience. On Sunday, I had emotional highs and lows, with the highs higher and the lows lower than I have experienced in a long

time. I came in feeling empty, rejected, sorry for my-self, of no use to anyone, blah, blah...

My strategy for the day? To meet with several patients who had said "no" to the offer of a chaplain visit. Professionally speaking, I wanted to learn to deal better with these situations—to get some sense of the nuance of how to proceed beyond the "no."

But, to be honest, I was feeling rejected emotionally in general and so figured "misery loves company." Might as well get some more rejection as long as I'm at it. Diving into pain has been a key learning method for me for a long time, at least that's how I justify such action. Another element of the strategy, at least with this patient, was to spend time with someone whose life might be feeling miserable because mine sure was. In effect, if I could get past the expected "no," I might get cheered up.

When I'm feeling bad, cheery people don't often help. I'd rather find someone who understands my pain because of their own. I wasn't going to share my pain with Lee—that I knew would be unprofessional. But as you see in C6, I ultimately confessed to him that I came in because I wanted some company. He didn't go anywhere with this confession—other than more lessons about dealing with women—but at least I felt I had made an honest disclosure to him. Just before I said this to him, he had complimented me, and I felt dishonest in accepting the compliment.

I wasn't there for altruistic reasons.

One other point of reference: I did try to start the day with some cheerfulness. There was a mom who had delivered a healthy baby via C-section but who needed a few extra days of recovery for herself. So in I walked, and there was the happy father, worn-out mother and good-looking baby. They all had just finished a photography session and that glow was still present. We chatted, said a prayer together, presenting one more picture-perfect moment of chaplain praying as the mom and dad held the baby close between them.

Leaving them, I felt like I was still being a professional, doing my job. Not bad. Actually, this was a test of one of my motivations in shifting from my night chaplain work into CPE. At night, I felt I worked easily, capable of being fully present to patients and their families. But in applying for CPE, I wanted to see how well I could perform under more difficult conditions, either because of a hectic day with multiple conflicting demands on my time or because I didn't feel like I was working at full strength. Like I said, not bad with this couple and baby. But I hadn't done the wallowing I wanted to do that day, and so I shifted over to my list of "no chaplain needed" patients.

Here's another thing I've learned in the course of developing this verbatim. The training of a priest in my lineage of Rinzai Zen Buddhism is meant to develop two abilities:

• *"To become one with"—assaulting a dualistic approach to reality*
• *"To take away fear" in others*

These phrases are sometimes used interchangeably, but this patient encounter suggests that they are not of the same order of ability. *"To become one with"* might be seen as an expectation of any well-trained priest, something I feel we should be able to take for granted when we encounter a Zen priest.

But the greatest need for this ability to take away fear lies in those circumstances where the fear is the greatest. This suggests training that lies beyond that of the priest. I've spoken before about the role of martial arts training in my lineage of Zen, and I have heard my teachers emphasize this role.

The contrast I experienced with Lee was an ability to become one with but not an ability to take away fear. With Lee, those were not interchangeable abilities. This was a man who knew fear intimately and who had learned to bluster, maneuver, strong-arm his way around it or through it. Survival. But his manner suggested a deep fear was still present. Perhaps a fear that someone would find his weaknesses. Perhaps a fear that his children would not respect him. Perhaps a fear that he would die with nothing to show for his life.

For me to be able to take that fear away, I would need to be able to meet Lee on his own ground, a ground where we both stood with no defensive weapons. I was able to come onto his ground, but I had done it with a trick. I had said that I was in the room to learn from him and so had placed myself deliberately in a submissive position. That was the humbling that he felt in me.

I could have shifted out of the position once we were well into the conversation, but I didn't. I'm not sure why. I think it is because I am still adapting to a newly-discovered sense in which chaplains heal spiritual illnesses. We don't just join the patient; we seek a form of cure. I don't own this challenge yet, though I am seeking ways to explore it.

Finally, I want to reflect on my feelings about the fact that I used this patient to ease my pain rather than seeking to ease his. I should feel unprofessional and embarrassed but to be honest, I don't. There was a sense of mutuality at least—he was using me as much as I was using him and that too could have been grounds for the respect we felt for each other.

But this taps into some old biases of mine regarding the work of physicians. I often asked medical students to reflect on their need for people to be sick. They act as if the needs are only one way—there is a patient who needs help and the physician is there to provide it. But without a sick patient, a doctor has no job, no income. More deeply, without sick patients, doctors cannot soothe that deep need they feel to be of service to others through medicine.

*This is a genuine need, sometimes eloquently ex-
pressed, but it is rarely examined as a selfish need
rather than an altruistic one.*
   End

As I mentioned before, when presenting verbatims in
our small group—three chaplain residents, myself and
our supervisor—we read them aloud, then solicited discussion. I finished reading this one about the man with
kidney cancer and then went silent, feeling proud of myself. After a pause, Linda stood up, walked over to the
open door to our seminar room, and closed it. She came
back, sat down, saying:

"I am furious. I can't believe you treated that man
that way. This sounds like a man who knows just about
every form of powerlessness there is—and he has just had
a visit from an arrogant white man who feels he has the
authority to take away the last bit of power he might
possess—the power to say who he wants to talk with and
who he doesn't. Who the hell do you think you are?"

Long pause. I asked what else she might have to say.
Linda had a lot else to say, taking me through all the
ways in which I did harm to this patient, then describing the way in which I had done harm to her. She knew
the ground she stood on, having lived a life with many
assaults on her own dignity and sense of power. She con-
cluded finally by saying, "I don't feel safe around you."

We were already far beyond our usual quitting time.
For the most part, Jeff and the two other chaplain resi-

dents had remained silent. I felt drained—one more time in my life when I have to deal with an angry woman. I quickly stopped trying to explain my actions, recognizing that nothing I was saying eased the conflict.

Even though I could understand the logic of Linda's analysis and commentary, I kept thinking, "But you weren't there. You didn't feel how the atmosphere shifted over the course of the conversation. Didn't you hear me read Lee's words, saying that he felt respected by my approach?"

I felt that I hadn't harmed Lee, but clearly I had harmed my relationship with my colleague Linda, a woman I had grown to love for her great spirit and open heart. This felt like the death of a relationship that Jeff had warned me about. And it felt horrible.

Once home that evening, I decided that the only way forward was to resign from the training program. Whether I was right or wrong was not the issue. My early concerns about myself as a dangerous learner had become real, and I couldn't justify staying in the program if Linda felt unsafe. For all the damage she had suffered from me, at least I could let her feel safe by removing myself from the program.

The letter was written and delivered to Jeff's inbox before he arrived the next morning. By prior arrangement, Linda was scheduled to be away for the day, so I felt that I at least had a day to wrap up my responsibilities on the hospital units assigned to me. But during a morning break, I saw Jeff and asked for time to talk. He had read my letter before we sat down together.

Jeff pointed out that many of Linda's emotional

triggers had been hit by this verbatim report and by my manner when presenting it. He seemed to accept that the two needs I had that day—my need for comfort and my need for learning to deal with patients who were declining spiritual care—were valid ones to learn about, but that I had mixed them up in working with this patient.

He asked why I hadn't come to him first before plunging into this learning. He spoke a bit about my manner in facing Linda's great anger, saying that my relative calmness and absence of self-defense was not an example of the ability to recognize anxiety in another person and not get caught up in it. If I had been in that state, I would have been able to see Linda's needs more clearly and attended to them in the moment. In other words, I had survived her anger but had not taken care of her.

Jeff said that it was unnecessary to resign from the program, that both Linda and I had a great deal to learn from our encounter and he would be responsible for our well-being, especially her need to feel safe. Beyond words, though, was a feeling that he knew acutely my sense of sadness and humiliation.

He went to his files and said that he had something to give me, pulling out an English translation of the poem "The Man Watching" by German writer Rainer Maria Rilke. The last three stanzas sank in the deepest:

What we choose to fight is so tiny!
What fights with us is so great!
If only we would let ourselves be dominated

as things do by some immense storm,
we would become strong too, and not need names.

When we win it's with small things,
and the triumph itself makes us small.
What is extraordinary and eternal
does not want to be bent by us.
I mean the Angel who appeared
to the wrestlers of the Old Testament:
when the wrestlers' sinews
grew long like metal strings,
he felt them under his fingers
like chords of deep music.

Whoever was beaten by this Angel
(who often simply declined the fight)
went away proud and strengthened
and great from that harsh hand,
that kneaded him as if to change his shape.
Winning does not tempt that man.
This is how he grows: by being defeated, decisively,
by constantly greater beings.
(translated by Robert Bly)

This poem was a gift, presented without commentary. "When we win it's with small things, and the triumph itself makes us small. What is extraordinary and eternal does not want to be bent by us." Here was a glimmer that vulnerability could be a form of strength. Was that possible?

A week later, we went through a long written and verbal evaluation halfway through this three-month CPE training. We evaluated each other as colleagues. We evaluated Jeff as our supervisor. We evaluated the training program. As you might imagine, we also evaluated ourselves.

I was still absorbing the impact of the previous week's struggle, especially confronting Linda's comment that I made her feel unsafe. I had been proud of my Zen "edge," the sense of unease that people sometimes felt around me. But I had gone too far without thinking about the impact of my risk-taking on others. I was still feeling numb and exhausted.

I did thoroughly answer all the questions on the evaluation checklist, but my answers felt academic. But there were cracks in my numbness when writing about Jeff as supervisor and about my "theological growth."

Jeff's strength is his ability to model behaviors that may best help us as chaplains, especially the ability to see through anxiety, in himself and in others. I like that everything is open for discussion and feel that he gives me a fair hearing. I like his attitude of giving "an ounce for an ounce; a pound for a pound." For the most part, I feel he has given me "a ton for a ton." I like the fact that we can approach supervision with our own agenda in mind—he helps me to build upon several elements of the CPE training as well as integrate them. The last three lines of the Rilke are especially meaningful:

Winning does not tempt that man.
This is how he grows: by being defeated,
  decisively,
by constantly greater beings.

*I do tend to seek out "constantly greater beings" and
for me, CPE is providing a strong example of that.
There is no "winning" here, but there most definitely
is "growing." And that defeat doesn't feel like defeat.*

Theologically, what was happening to me? One way to
answer was to look at what was happening to my breath
and posture, my physicality as a chaplain, core elements
of the theology of a Zen priest. I was pleased to find that
those were holding up much better than expected. The
work was physically demanding and could pull us several different directions at once. Nonetheless, for the most
part when I checked my breath and posture, they seemed
optimized for the situation.

This connection between physicality and theology
seems far-fetched but it is worth exploring. For example,
when attending to a dying patient and their family, when
there is no useful thing to do, I found myself naturally
working for the optimal breath and posture of "being."
That meant there was a felt sense, a visceral sense. What
use of breath and posture makes me most available to them?

This is manual labor. I'm finding there was natural
feedback from the atmosphere of the room or the atti-

tude of the patient that told me whether or not I was on the right track. There is indeed a physicality of being. And it can be deepened on the spot, as needed.

Perhaps the best example happened when I was attending to a family and a patient who had just died. Out of respect for the family, the door to his room was kept closed. When I returned from taking a call at the nursing station, it felt appropriate to knock before entering, given the ongoing grief of his two daughters in the room. As I began the first of three knocks, I felt gravity sink through my body in a certain way. I had a momentary flash that there might be only one way to knock in the face of such solemnity.

8.
Nothing special.
We get them all the time.

L ast week I had felt thoroughly beaten by Linda, by myself, by Rilke's sinewy angel, the one who "does not want to be bent by us." And I found, strangely enough, that defeat made me feel more alive. This coming week, that liveliness began to work.

The first sign of this new capacity to be with others was with a young woman in the intensive care unit. I had met Gillian during her last visit to this hospital, which had been for a heroin overdose. She survived that overdose, but not the next one. Now she was being kept "alive" while being evaluated as a potential organ donor.

Rather than focusing on Gillian for my next verbatim assignment, I examined an encounter with Grace, an ICU nurse anchoring Gillian's care. My conversation with the veteran nurse took place during a short visit.

Additional Factual Information:

Gillian arrived at the Emergency Room last Sunday morning, following an overdose of heroin. Declared brain dead at 12:44 p.m., she continued receiving life support while the organ transplant team evaluated the suitability of several of her organs for transplant.

Ten days ago, this patient had been admitted to the ICU following a heroin overdose, was stabilized and then transferred to the 6th floor, where I first met her and her mother, Cathy. When meeting her on her initial stay on the 6th floor, my impression was of a young woman who had no interest whatsoever in ending her drug use. Pleasant to talk to, Gillian showed little awareness of the dangers of her addiction.

According to her mother Cathy, Gillian had long been a rebel, both at home and at school. She was strongly attached to her father, though her parents had divorced 14 years ago. Roughly one year ago, her father committed suicide, supposedly in despair over an inability to control his alcoholism, a struggle compounded by a bi-polar condition.

According to Cathy, Gillian had begun using heroin before her father died—perhaps contributing to his despair—but she used it more heavily after his death.

At the time of her overdose, Gillian was living

with her boyfriend. It was determined that he had injected the dose of heroin that caused her latest overdose, and he was now in jail, waiting to find if he would be held responsible for her death and charged with homicide.

Cathy could talk about this boyfriend in a fairly level voice, saying, "He must have done that injection at her request. I don't believe he would have just come up to her in her sleep and stuck the needle in. But I don't know...."

Over the hours I spent with Cathy, she was distraught but also somewhat detached from the full pain of having her daughter die this way. As we stood beside Gillian's bed, she said, "It's funny. Look at her. This is the best she has looked in a long time. When she was using heroin a lot, she would get so skinny and have those dark pouches beneath her eyes. But her last visit here really fattened her up. Just look at that face...." Yes, Gillian had a beautiful face.

When I left the ICU at 4:30 p.m. that Monday, Cathy was explaining to a member of the transplant team that she was eager to have her daughter donate organs so that "something of her lives on." But she wanted to know when during the donation process her daughter would actually die.

The transplant team member coldly replied, "Well, she is dead already. That happened yesterday."

Cathy knew that Gillian's skin was still warm,

and her face had color. Cathy could see her daughter's chest rising and falling as her breathing was
done by a machine. So how could Gillian be dead?

Cathy wanted to know when those signs of life
would end if they decided her daughter's organs
could be put to use. She asked me to be in the op-
erating room when that happened. I told her how
sorry I was that this would not be possible, and that
if Gillian went to surgery that night, Cathy would
be saying goodbye to her daughter in her ICU room.
I told Cathy I would be sure that the night chaplain
was available as needed.

Finally, there is one other bit of background
information. Grace, the ICU nurse, told a night
chaplain that there had been twelve deaths in this
hospital's ICU over the past month, an unusually
high number. Some of these cases have been difficult
in terms of family dynamics, and Grace had been
actively part of several of those cases.

Plans:

On Tuesday morning, I received the news from the
night chaplain that Gillian had not gone to surgery
as planned. Her organs were declared unsuitable
for use. Once support was withdrawn Monday evening, Cathy was able to grasp that her daughter
was indeed dead. Cathy had previously told a social
worker that she didn't have the money for a funeral
for her daughter, so it was unclear what happened

to Gillian's body.

Having heard this news, I went to the ICU with a vague desire to see what might remain of this young woman. Most likely Gillian's body would not still be in a bed, but maybe there would be a lingering feeling of her amidst the machines and tubes.

Observations:

In the ICU, Gillian's room was empty. It had already been readied for a new patient. Sunlight came in the window in a way that made the room feel new and fresh. There was no feeling of the patient left behind, other than my own sadness.

I said hello to the unit clerk and looked around the front area of the ICU, noticing there was little staff movement, probably because there were so few ICU patients that day. I was turning to leave when I noticed Grace, the veteran nurse who had been working with Gillian and Cathy on Monday. Since I had not been there when the ventilator had been pulled, I wanted to hear the end of Gillian's story.

During our Monday conversations when I had been asking for updates regarding the evaluation of the patient's organs, Grace had maintained a formal and professional manner. She provided the facts, then turned away. She showed no interest in lingering. During our Tuesday encounter, she maintained the same affect, willing to answer my questions but coldly.

The visit:

C1: *[catching her eye] I'm just checking in about our patient from yesterday. I've seen the notes. [Notice that I didn't greet this nurse by name]*

N1: *Yeah?*

C2: *I saw that organ donation was not possible, so that meant her mom could get some closure here [meaning that she could be present when support was withdrawn].*

N2: *Yes, it went well.*

C3: *So, what happened regarding a funeral home? I know the mom said she couldn't afford a funeral.*

N3: *Right. She couldn't decide what to do so we never called anyone. [So far, this nurse's manner seems to ask, "Are you done with the questions yet?" This had also been her demeanor the day before.]*

C4: *So, where is Gillian now? In the morgue? [I think I was asking this because I wanted to see her again, if possible. Like Cathy, I could grasp the "brain death" intellectually, but felt another need to fully understand Gillian was actually dead, not coming back.]*

N4: *No, she went to autopsy.*

C5: *Is that done here or at the university?*

N5: *The university I think, so that's where she must be now. They'll have to figure out the funeral arrangements. [Finally, Grace is slowing down a bit and not being quite so dismissive.]*

C6: *That's got to be rough on her mom. Was it her desire to have an autopsy?*

N6: *No, the medical examiner's...*

C7: *Because of the heroin...*

N7: *No, because of the homicide. [This last word "homicide" was said with unusual emphasis. Spoken still in the flat emotionless way everything else had been said by her, but with enough breath behind "homicide" for me to feel the pain behind this word.]*

C8: *Right, I heard that. Well, you all have seen a lot of overdoses lately.*

N8: *Nothing special. We get them all the time. Two more found outside the doors of the mall this morning.*

C9: *No [with a shake of my head]—I hadn't heard that.*

N9: *Well, listen to the news! [This whole phrase was uttered with much more emphasis than the earlier word "homicide." I felt that she was angry with me for not being fully informed.]*

C10: *OK. Thank you for all your help yesterday. [Notice that there is enough room between N9 and C10 to drive a truck.]*

Analysis — the Nurse

I have some self-identification with Grace. We share a sense of toughness, perhaps protecting ourselves from expressing strong feeling, but I'm finding it strange to be admitting this sense of "protection" of myself.

With so little understanding of Grace's life and values, it feels wrong to address elements of her psychological well-being. As I wrote, however, in my verbatim about Cass and Alex, I might be best able to help her if I had a better awareness of her coping mechanisms. How do they serve her? How do they harm her? Grace has lasted a long time in her job, so she may not be at risk of burnout. It is hard to imagine she hasn't seen similar stretches of stressful patients and deaths before.

Looking at our short conversation today, I was struck by the strength of her feelings when she said the word "homicide" and then her command, "Listen to the news!" They felt all the angrier because of the contrast with the level tones of the rest of her words. Grace was clearly affected by this Gillian's death but was not going to readily admit that.

Analysis — the Chaplain

Looking back at this encounter as I write this, I feel that I went to the ICU that morning looking for a sense of closure for the strong emotions experienced the day before when spending hours with Gillian and her mother. I felt a great sense of sadness at the loss of this young woman's life.

Sadness that Cathy should feel that her daughter's death was inevitable, given her heroin addiction. Sadness that a mother should feel her daugh-

ter's heroin use may have contributed to the suicide of her own father. And that a mother should know her daughter's boyfriend is being charged with homicide because of his role in her death. That a mother should worry that her one remaining child, a son in high school, may not know how to handle the loss of his father and his sister in the same year. That a mother should look so thin and frail herself, unable to absorb all that was happening, saying with no conviction whatsoever, "Well, in the end I'll be OK."

My sadness was compounded by the feelings of loss I had been experiencing these past several weeks. I became aware of these losses as part of a cascade of losses stretching back decades: the loss of my first marriage, the loss of a life with my children when they were growing up, the loss of good friends when I moved from place to place, the loss of a normal set of neuromuscular reflexes for my youngest son, the loss of an academic promotion after working so hard as a faculty member at the medical school, the loss of the business partnership I had formed with my son when we first moved to Wisconsin. I'm guessing there are more losses in my life that I have yet to bring back to the surface. But the sadness of loss looms large in my life.

That awareness is new. For the past twenty years, perhaps longer, my basic stance in life has been, "I will not feel the sadness of loss." I had mas-

tered this skill of avoidance. It is strange to look at this in the context of hospital chaplain work because we are faced with loss all the time.

That brings to mind a Japanese phrase, "aware no mono." It translates to something like "an awareness of the fleeting nature of things," like a cherry blossom, a love affair, a life. Things that once gone cannot be recovered, so one must savor them in the moment, savor them deeply while not forgetting that, ultimately, they are fleeting.

I see where some of my deep love of Japan comes from, and also see that I have not fully absorbed the lesson of "aware no mono." Many times my losses caught me by surprise rather than feeling inevitable. I thought that friendships, vacations with my children, meaningful work as a medical school faculty member, would last forever. In Buddhism, such illusions are "attachment," the cause of all suffering.

But suffering doesn't make attachments bad. Some attachments are natural, like the love of a father for his children. They are part of our fabric as human beings. And some attachments may be voluntary, perhaps something like my love for the woods and meadows of our home and Dojo.

Pastoral opportunity
Clearly, there was an opportunity for pastoral care of ICU nurse Grace to be found in that gap

between her vehement "Well, listen to the news" when talking about recent heroin overdoses and my response, "Thank you for your help yesterday." I didn't take the opportunity to explore Grace's re-action. At the time, I didn't even recognize that I could have.

Like me, Grace may have developed her tough-ness to avoid the sadness of loss. Understandable because the nature of her work is to attempt to save patients' lives, even under the most difficult con-ditions. I would imagine that she has more than mastered the skill of avoidance. So how could I pro-vide spiritual care to her? I imagine that in no way would she grant me much credibility as a loss coun-selor in the ICU context.

I needed to join her in her protective posture, but what would this look like? Perhaps I could ap-proach Grace and say that, as a chaplain in train-ing, I noticed how I avoid feeling sadness of loss. I would say that, given her setting for patient care, she must face loss all day long and that I would like to learn how she deals with it. Ask Grace to teach me.

End

My learning during the six weeks that led to this en-counter felt ferocious, nothing held back. But reading this verbatim more than five years after these events, it is embarrassing to read how little care I provided to Grace.

I was attending to my needs for closure in this conversation with her and had nothing to offer Grace despite her veiled revelation of strong emotion surrounding this Gillian's death. That is hard to admit, but true.

Still, in saying these things, I recognize the attitude of a first-year medical student after their first attempt at history-taking with a real patient. I've watched them emerge from the examination room and lament to fellow students how poorly they had just handled the interview. "Duh! I never even thought to ask him about smoking. How stupid!"

We're talking about an incredibly sophisticated human skill: gathering all possible information from someone during a discussion while simultaneously making it a therapeutic interaction. In the context of Japanese forms of craft, there is a phrase that roughly translates as "Do it 10,000 times; then you can begin to learn." Whether making ceramics or flower arrangements or practicing sword cuts, there is a clear recognition that the body and the senses are being trained far more profoundly than the mind. And the only way for that to happen is for exhaustive repetition, doing the work of finding what's most natural.

The same is true with patient encounters. If I were to have written one hundred verbatims, the recent ones might feel more caring of the patient. If I was writing after forty years of hospital chaplaincy with tens of thousands of encounters with patients, there might be no sense of a chaplain present, but a patient well cared for.

That is my ideal of chaplaincy: a chaplain without ego and a patient healed. In this nurse encounter, I am still a beginner, focused more on my own learning than on the needs of the person in front of me.

9.
I have lost so much in my life.

One of the most iconic images of Buddhism is that of Kannon (in Japanese) or Kuan-yin (in Mandarin), the Bodhisattva of Compassion. This figure is most often depicted as a woman, with a gentle posture and a half-smile. To the degree that any of us associate compassion with our own mother—the loving embrace, the forgiving smile—this depiction brings comfort to Buddhists and non-Buddhists alike.

I want to explore this Buddhist ideal of compassion from several different directions, based on my own Zen training and my experiences to date as a CPE intern. As you might expect, the Zen perspective of compassion is not quite as simple.

I remember a conversation with my 85-year-old-mother a few weeks ago. I had asked for time alone with her to discuss a heartfelt struggle I've been having, and the result was a remarkable experience.

I started the conversation with an aged woman seated across from me, a woman with trouble breathing because of her COPD, with deep pains in her ankles and knees anytime she walks, and with the heartache of living with my father as he starts losing his memory.

But as we talked more, I felt the years drop off her shoulders, watched her eyes sharpen and facial wrinkles smooth over, and heard her lean into my woes with all the love and caring I have ever experienced from her.

So, yes, my image of compassion starts with my own mother. Acceptance, understanding, forgiveness, sharing, strength, love, protection—all these things I felt from her. When I first sat down with her, I wasn't expecting her responses. I thought she might express disappointment, confusion, hurt. But there were none of that. Her compassion felt like an unexpected or undeserved gift.

But compassion knows no gender. Here are two examples of a masculine form of compassion. It was Saturday evening and, as the cook for an intensive three days of Zen training, I was supervising the serving of dinner. Seated on the floor were ten people, each of them in front of a low table holding their bowls and food. The tables were arranged in a U-shape, with the group's young meditation leader and a senior teacher from Hawaii seated at the head table.

Late afternoon sun was coming in on their faces, one

that of a 30-year-old-man and the other that of a 68-year-old-man. The face of the young man showed the sharpness but weariness you might see in the face of a surgeon after performing a ten-hour procedure on a patient.

The face of the older man showed a lifetime of caring for the well-being of others. He comes to our Wisconsin Dojo twice each year for four weeks, moving slowly and easily throughout the day, keeping an eye out for anything that needs attending to, whether it is the fire heating the outdoor Japanese bath, fixing a broken chainsaw, playing his Japanese flute in the twilight for the owls, teaching a young woman the meaning of sound. He doesn't have the strength of the younger man but has a depth that comes from a lifetime of setting the needs of others before his own.

Although I started with the image of my mother as the embodiment of compassion, these two faces from the world of Zen come closer to my own understanding of the word. I will explain this understanding through another scene from that weekend's training.

We were in the meditation period following dinner. People had been sitting motionless for long stretches of time and their legs hurt, their knees hurt. And still they sat motionless.

In the midst of the silence, the young leader stood and picked up a piece of wood, a *keisaku*, shaped something like a sword but with a broad flat face. He walked down the line of students, stopping before one of them, bowing, then kneeling into a posture that one uses in sword training.

The student, sitting likewise, bowed and bent forward, his arms pulled tightly across his chest. Suddenly, the keisaku came down with a crack. Three times, the student's back was struck on one side, then three times on the other. The sound echoed.

People have heard of this use of a stick in Zen meditation, but why and how it is used is often misunderstood. I call this striking an act of deep compassion but recognize that I must explain this clearly. When done correctly, the feeling after the strike is tremendous clarity. Pain disappears, one's vision opens widely, the body becomes wonderfully erect, feeling the full force of gravity on your bones and muscle. Thoughts stop, not just for the student struck but also for everyone in the room.

What has happened? As one meditates, the physical work is to let all things, body and mind, settle, viscerally settle. But pain can be a counter-active force to this settling. It rises up, filling the head, but also filling the sets of muscles lying along the spine in the upper back, causing those muscles to tense. When those same back muscles are properly struck, that tenseness disappears and gravity can work once again. And, given the quality of the sound of the smack, each person in the room feels it as well.

To be compassionate in this way takes a high degree of training. If there is any sense of holding back, any fear of hurting the person being struck, any doubts in the mind of the meditation leader, the striking is not an act of compassion, even if well-intentioned. Instead, it hurts physically and brings out feelings of strong anger in the person struck.

The training to become such a leader is not just learning how to swing a sword. It is shugyo, the Japanese word that imperfectly translates as "spiritual forging," forging in the sense of having one's spirit, one's identity, plunged into fire, pounded into shape, plunged into cold water—these acts, over and over and over again. In this sense the compassion comes out of that forging.

Coming back to the phrase "Bodhisattva of Compassion," here is a dictionary definition of a bodhisattva: "In Mahayana Buddhism [a very broad category that includes Zen Buddhism], a bodhisattva is a being who seeks Buddhahood through the systematic practice of the perfect virtues but renounces complete entry into nirvana until all beings are saved." What is nirvana? The same source describes it as "oneness with the absolute... dwelling in the experience of the absolute...freedom from attachment to illusions, affects and desires."

Why delay entrance into nirvana? Compassion, emerging from insight and wisdom. A bodhisattva takes on the suffering of all other beings, saying in effect, "I'm willing to suffer if it will ease your suffering."

For this particular bodhisattva, the Sanskrit name is Avalokiteshvara. A translation of this name is sometimes rendered as "Regarder of the Cries of the World." This phrasing means a great deal to me because it depicts compassion as a visceral experience—the sensory ability

and physical strength to hear all the cries of the world—
and not as an abstract virtue. My hearing—actually, all
my senses—sharpens when my breath and my posture
are developed to the point where my ordinary sense of
self falls away.

The defining sutra for this bodhisattva is The Sutra of
the Lotus Flower of the Wonderful Law. Chapter XXV is
entitled "The All-Sidedness of the Bodhisattva Regarder
of the Cries of the World," and it starts like this:

> *At that time the Bodhisattva Infinite Thought rose
> up from his seat, and baring his right shoulder
> and folding his hands toward the Buddha, spoke
> thus: "World-honored one! For what reason is the
> Bodhisattva Avalokitsevara named Regarder of the
> Cries of the World?"*
>
> *The Buddha answered the Bodhisattva Infinite
> Thought: "Good son! If there be countless hundred
> thousand myriad kotis of living beings suffering
> from pain and distress who hear of this Bodhisat-
> tva, Regarder of the Cries of the World, and with
> all their mind call upon his name, the Bodhisattva,
> Regarder of the Cries of the World, will instantly
> regard their cries, and all of them will be delivered.*
>
> *If there be any who keep the name of that
> Bodhisattva, Regarder of the Cries of the World,
> though they fall into a great fire, the fire will not
> be able to burn them, by virtue of the supernatural
> power of that bodhisattva's majesty. If any, carried*

away by a flood, call upon his name, they will im-
mediately reach the shallows...

For many Buddhists, this passage suggests that when they are in distress or danger, there is a power to whom they can pray for comfort and deliverance from suffering. I can acknowledge the power of this comfort across thousands of years and millions of lives.

But from the Zen perspective, there is a problem with this interpretation. The passage says, "If there be...living beings suffering from pain and distress," as if there is such a sub-category of human beings. With the Four Noble Truths, the Buddha teaches that, because of the dualistic way in which we view the world, it is natural for all human beings to suffer, not just some human beings.

This dualism leads to attachment—to wealth, friends, beliefs. And attachment by nature leads to suffering, because we are trying to stop the inevitable process of change. For me, this means that Kannon perceives all human beings simply as we are, hearing the sounds we make as we face a deluded world of our own creation. All living beings are perceived simultaneously, as they are. This is a very different image of the role of Kannon from the more usual one in which she/he simply answers the prayers of the afflicted. "To hear all"—no different from feeling all, witnessing all—is a far more profound view of compassion to me.

The sutra goes on to say that Kannon makes fearless

those in anxiety and distress. Again, "those in anxiety and distress" is not a sub-category of living beings. It means all living beings. This gift of fearlessness is a direct result of a simultaneous perception of all suffering; meaning perception of the natural state of all living beings.

Given all this, when asked, "What is the meaning of compassion?" I answer as deeply as I can, "The gift of fearlessness." Phrased another way, when capable of such perception, the natural result is compassion.

I can't emphasize this enough: compassion is a deeply physical experience.

Circling back, this physical experience is the natural end result of shugyo, spiritual forging. I say "end result" as if there were an end, but actually the training never ends.

Most people begin their Zen training to ease pain in their lives—emotional pain, physical pain, psychological pain. For me, it was the pain of experiencing a huge chasm between myself and others. But with time and effort, I found that the more profound work was to ease the pain in someone else's life.

I don't have to try doing that; it just happens when the physical sensation of compassion is found. And that compassion becomes "found" as a dualistic conception of self and other begins to dissolve. Said another way, compassion is not delivered from one person to another the way you might hand over a cool glass of water. It is a physical experience, perceived as two or more people are joined in their suffering.

So finally, here's the last shift of scene: to the ICU,

where I spent many hours with Cathy after her daughter overdosed on heroin. In what way did I bring compassion to this mother and daughter?

The honest answer is that I don't know. But certainly something happened as we spent time together, both while talking and sitting silently. The physical work that I felt myself doing was twofold: filling this fragile mother with my strength and entering into her sadness. I say "physical" because my work involved adjusting my breath and posture so that as much strength as possible was being given, and to keep adjusting breath and posture so that I could feel her sadness as much as possible.

There is another way in which this is physical work. All the time that I am deepening breath and posture, I was being challenged by the sadness Cathy kept expressing, some of it from long ago, some freshly-delivered as we sat through the day.

One after the other, Cathy's losses were hard to take emotionally. Hard to take because they triggered my own experiences of sadness and loss. I felt each of her sadnesses strike my body as I learned them. I felt each of my sadnesses in my body as they were triggered, and all the while I was supposed to be optimizing the use of my breath and posture to give her strength, to give her myself.

After seeing another patient, I returned and found Cathy seated in the ICU waiting room. She was ending a phone call as I stood in front of her. She said in a flat voice, "That was the District Attorney. Gillian's boyfriend is being charged with her murder."

It took all my strength to let this news wash through me, leaving me steady and not rocked back on my heels. And yet Cathy had to hear this news, and I had to keep filling her with strength and to be completely present to her, and not get caught in my own anger at Gillian's boyfriend.

This was what I call "facing suffering"—the physical act of letting someone's suffering flood through you, feeling it fully, but not letting it wash you away.

Overall, I've described three forms of compassion: the love of a parent, the clarity of a swordsman or swordswoman, and the ability to face suffering without crumbling. I want to talk about another form of compassion: the data-gathering that happens for me in patient encounters.

Data-gathering helps me get more specific in the care I provide. It may be a cold-sounding term, but it refers back to the act of precise perception, or "regarding," embedded in the Sanskrit name of the Bodhisattva of Compassion.

One by-product of Zen training in breath and posture over long periods of time is that your senses sharpen. I'm not always conscious of what detail my senses pick up from an encounter, but after the fact I may find myself full of a sense of richness.

Above, I wrote: "All living beings are perceived simultaneously, simply as they are." In this spirit, I returned to Gillian's mother as her daughter lay so still in the ICU.

Cathy was incredibly thin. It was not a sickly thinness or a diet-based thinness, but a brittle kind of thinness.

There was a stiffness to her movements that made her seem like she was wearing a shell. It was a shell with little room inside. The walls of the shell were close together.

I told myself, "There's no life inside her. It has been sucked out of her and as that happened, the walls of her shell started to collapse."

I noticed fresh scabs on her face—one right down the middle of her chin and several on her forehead. And she held her body such that her torso, head and neck were tilted about fifteen degrees off a vertical axis, bent toward her right side. Finally, there was little resonance in Cathy's voice—meaning the sounds were produced more in her throat than in her abdomen. The muscles of her chest and abdomen were tensed.

I sensed a woman with little resilience who was being physically twisted by years of suffering. Asked about the scabs on her face, Cathy said that she had been so lost in her thoughts that she had walked into a closed door. Given this state, her capacity for absorbing all the emotions and feelings surrounding her daughter and son were limited.

I felt respectful of that, knowing how I have sought numbness when first encountering great pain, letting that numbness protect me until something within is ready to feel again. But I was worried that she might not be able to come out of her numbness spontaneously—it might last a long time. My work with Cathy—whether we were talking or silent, with Gillian or eating lunch downstairs—was to breathe life into her. Not too much, but just enough so that she would have a sense of her own body again, ready to feel when she was ready.

We were now at the end of the week and it was time for my sixth supervisory conference, a chance to reflect on the onslaught of learning over the past two weeks. Jeff felt my new vulnerability as I dropped the stance of feeling no sadness from loss. Jeff and I spoke of the power of vulnerability—of setting down the sword. We talked about the ways in which my vulnerability could help me with patients who were still relatively closed up.

I work well with patients who are wide open in their suffering. I jump right in. But now I wanted to see how I could get to the suffering any of us experience with illness, whether suffering is on the surface or not.

I remembered the fear and helplessness I experienced when I had meningitis years ago, and how resistant I had been to taking care of myself once I began recovering. Some part of me had been saying "I will not feel this fear, this helplessness." Now I was feeling a more peaceful confidence of wholeness, my power and my weakness were together.

My learning was soaking into my bones and not just my head. I could work with patients whose suffering was not obvious, as compared to those I had earlier called "train wrecks." I had thought that I had some kind of gift for dealing with those difficult patients. Instead, I was being lazy, finding that I worked best with those whose suffering was obvious. This new learning was that power comes from wholeness, with both my strengths and my weaknesses working together.

The test of this learning came later that afternoon, as I visited Mrs. Baker, an elderly woman in her room on one of the regular medical units. I had no special mission with this visit, other than rounding out my day's work.

Mrs. Baker looked like so many elderly women I've seen in this hospital: clear-eyed, calm, alert. I introduced myself and asked how she was doing. There was a long pause in that late afternoon light, tears came to her eyes, and she said, "I have lost so much in my life." I was stunned in a way I had not experienced before with a patient. Her words, her emotions, seemed to come out of thin air.

As Mrs. Baker spoke, I felt all my losses in the room as well. It struck me: because I know my losses, she can know hers. It was the simplest thing in the world.

This must be what it means to be the therapeutic instrument that I wanted to my students to understand during my time as a medical school faculty member. In a fraught situation, there may be nothing to do, and everything to be. But that being must be self-aware.

Self-awareness is the point of chaplain training.

10.
Seeing the pebble
clearly on the bottom.

How do I now describe the aftermath of those weeks of crisis and drama? As my work shifted, it was as if there was less and less of me present and more and more of the people I encountered.

I've presented several cases in which there appeared to be drama, conflict, difficulties, but looking at them now it is clear the drama presented was more within me than in the situation itself. That doesn't mean it was any less serious or painful for those involved. It means that I was starting to see my own role in the drama.

An example where that clarity was resoundingly obvious came in the form of a Critical Incident Report: a CPE format for reporting and reflecting on a meaningful encounter with a patient, a family member, a colleague, or a member of the medical staff. It is meant to be short and quick, a more immediate capture than a verbatim. The first one that I wrote came after the weekly staff meeting in which there was review of patients who had been in the hospital more than fifteen days.

There were about a dozen people present at that meeting, and we had finished discussing the patients who were formally up for review. The meeting leader invited comments on anyone else we thought might be important for the assembled group to know about.

There was a long pause... then Jen Nehls, one of the social workers, spoke up, mentioning a woman who died last night. This woman and her two sons were familiar to many of us in the room. Jen was especially moved by the character of the two sons and the degree of caring they demonstrated to their mother. She spoke of their open souls, saying:

Looking at them was like looking into a mountain stream and seeing the pebbles clearly on the bottom.

The room became still. The air was cleared. For a moment, the rest of us in the room could look through that same mountain stream to the pebbles on the bottom. Some people looked down at the table, some looked with admiration at Jen. Some people looked into the distance, as if finding their own memories of working with these two sons.

I was startled by her words. Jen had been talking

about the sons in general, describing how devoted they were to their mother. But suddenly here was unexpected poetry.

This image felt so true. I felt happy/sad that these two son's disabilities—we had surmised that they had Asperger's Syndrome—may have given them this rare clarity of character, an ability to be open with their feelings and emotions. It made me think of my son Sam, someone whom I feel has something of this same clarity. There are times when it feels otherworldly.

I felt wonder that this social worker, someone that I had worked with and whom I admired for her gentle toughness, could suddenly bring to the group a feeling of love for these two men. I felt jealous that Jen could see them more clearly than me. I could not have spoken of them so lovingly, especially in this setting, with people from several different professions. I was humbled.

This was a highlight moment during my CPE training, a moment that cut through layers of "hospitalness." In my work here, I continually strived to excavate down to the humanity of the patient and the family. But I treat it like work—hard work—and forget that such perception of others is available most all the time with most all patients, family members and staff to any of us.

These last few days had felt strange. I felt disconnected from myself and others. I felt like I've been willingly holding onto a live electric wire for a long time—letting the juice course through me—but have finally, somehow, let something go. It felt like I let down a force field unconsciously held in place, a sword stance that was unrelenting, a way of being, I felt unplugged, a bit empty, unsure.

Yet in the midst of these observations, a flash of poetry came from an unexpected place, from an unexpected source. I considered that perhaps this way of perceiving could become part of a new way of being for me. Not pumping adrenaline all the time but remaining open to the beauty available from most anyone, most any time. I felt like a newborn, looking out at the world.

I could also feel how proud I had become of the work I was doing to help any and all of us in the hospital become human. If a patient encounter was hard work, and I succeeded, then I must be doing something worthwhile.

It was something like the self-identity I crafted while at the medical school in Hawaii. There would be a committee meeting, everyone would introduce themselves, including their roles at the school. It was easy to say "a medical educator in the Department of Family Medicine," but if I was feeling annnoyed in the face of perceived numbness in those present—patients being discussed as objects rather than human beings—I might say, "I'm not a physician, but I am the one professional human being on the faculty." Nervous laughter would follow.

This encounter with Jen was a reminder that humanity was all around me, ever present, not something needing excavation by a Zen guy.

This insight was a variation on my recognition that labeling Cass and Alex—the angry wife and jokester husband—as dysfunctional was not as helpful as asking why they had chosen their own particular coping mechanisms. By seeing them as whole and complete initially, I could be more nuanced when looking at the ways in which elements of their behavior hurt them more than helped.

I was increasingly watching for the triggers that might kick me into unnecessary intensity. That had been such a deep part of my identity, part of the logger, builder, swordsman, pioneer in the wilderness persona that I had become in Wisconsin as I built our Zen Dojo.

I had come back to the Midwest after twenty-two years in Hawaii for two reasons: to be closer to my aging parents and to create a Zen training center. To teach Zen in the manner that felt most natural, I wanted lots of land with hills, lots of hardwood trees and no existing buildings. For better or for worse, I wanted to build from the ground up, using our own wood, such that our buildings would "teach" Zen as much as I did.

That vision fit a need in my identity—a Bowie knife between my teeth as I survived blizzards. If the conditions were tough, I must be tough. If the oak trees felled were big and strong, I must be big and strong. In effect, I was creating a place where the environment matched my sense of identity. Now, with my patients, with my hospital colleagues, I was starting to learn that I could use that toughness and intensity only when needed. It was no longer permanently turned on.

This was similar to something learned early in my Zen training. I had grown up as a smart kid—not much of an athlete, but I was intelligent. I used that intelligence to navigate my way in the world. Doing that, I came to believe that the world inside my head was the same as the world outside. My divorce was the experience that painfully showed me that was untrue. What I thought of our marriage and what my wife thought of our marriage were very different.

That was the point at which my Zen training became deadly serious. If my thoughts did not mirror reality, then how do I live? If my intelligence didn't make my Zen training more effective, what good was it? I came to realize that I was not my thoughts. I came to see my intelligence as a specialized tool, one to be used when appropriate, set aside when of no use. The phrase I used to describe this was that "a good surgeon doesn't use a scalpel to pick her nose." I had learned this early about my intelligence, but I hadn't learned it about my intensity. In my chaplain training, I finally did.

Another deepening realization for me was the physical nature of the chaplain work. This arose when my colleague Collin was describing his frustration while working with the family of an elderly woman in the ICU.

The elderly patient and her bed had been wheeled out of her room, taken elsewhere for some sort of procedure. Seven or eight adult family members were left in the room, the setting that Collin stepped into. He described walking into the center of the room, introducing himself, asking how the family members were doing, and getting no response. He was known to be an effective chaplain and was confused as to why this encounter had not gone well.

I asked if I could stage a role-play as a way of helping him gain insight. Jeff and Collin said "OK," so I had our CPE team sit in a circle roughly the size of that grouping of family with nothing in the middle.

Collin stepped into that circle, introduced himself, and then waited to see what sort of conversation he could elicit.

Those of us in the circle stayed silent. Collin stood uncomfortably, all six and a half feet of him. Finally, he moved to the side of one of us, and knelt. And then a conversation could begin.

When Collin entered that patient room and stood in the middle, he stood right where this patient had been before she was taken out. That act must have caused anger, that a stranger would presume to occupy the place where their mother, aunt, friend had been just minutes before. By shifting to the periphery of the room, he got closer to joining the family members in their sadness and concern—physically closer—and no longer taking the place of the patient.

Again, my point is that there is a physicality to our work. How we stand in relationship to another person affects the quality of the conversation. I'm not just talking about the distance between us or the angle of our bodies relative to each other. As I stand, how I take gravity through my body and down to the ground has a large effect on my breathing and my state of awareness. Both of those things very much affect the quality of the conversation.

Not long after this role play, there was another supervisory conference with Jeff. We discussed a question from Scott, asked during the previous day's small group seminar: "So, Gordon, how is that Zen thing working out?"

I can't remember the context of the question nor could I speak to a reason for the seeming aggression embedded in the question. Jeff described to me during our conference how he had gone on high alert hearing Scott, wondering if I would take the bait.

I'm not sure why, but I chose to answer the question as asked, not the challenge implied. Jeff was surprised but pleased that I did not feel a reflexive need to engage in the fight.

I also wanted to describe something of the rich emotions I was now experiencing as I continued to explore losses I had experienced in my life. I flashed back to a forty-year-old memory from my first trip to Japan. I was on a small island in the south of Japan, watching a small fishing boat pull out from harbor, watching a father on the dock as his teenage son, also a fisherman, headed out to sea.

This memory of the longing between them was so vivid, remembering the sense of touch in their hands as they held two ends of a long paper streamer until it finally broke as the boat got too far from the dock. That sensation of "Please don't go, please don't go," all the while knowing that the going must be. And then the break in the paper streamer, showing that the going is real, and all the longing in the world can't stop it from happening.

Jeff said, "Gordon, you really feel things deeply..." That is true. I want to feel all things clearly, but I know there is a price that I pay. My chaplain training was a time to come to grips with my sensitivity to the world around me. If that sensitivity simply led to reactions—reacting to the challenge in Scott's question—my life was not my own. I would always be swimming in the currents of the waters surrounding me. But by recognizing that I could have all my feelings and sensitivity without becoming victim to them, I felt more whole.

Like my intelligence, like my intensity, I could have my sensitivity without being victim to it. When I said that there was a "price to pay," I meant that when I feel things acutely, there is a sensation of rawness that comes with it, not always welcome, but necessary.

11.
Oh, is that so?

fter ten weeks of CPE training, we were asked to articulate the nature of "pastoral care" that our work with patients had evoked. The challenge, however, was that in my training as a Zen priest, there was no concept such as pastoral care. The only instructions we were given about the work of a Zen priest were "to become one with" and "take away fear."

In my report, I chose to answer the a more literal question: "What does a Zen guy have to offer patients in a hospital?" By showing the nature of my training, I wanted to show the grounds of my perspective on patient care as I function as a Zen chaplain. Fearing that I might get too abstract in exploring the question, I decided to shape the essay as a letter to Jeff:

November 9

Dear Jeff,

Pastoral care is a huge subject, but a welcome one since it prompts me to integrate my CPE experiences with things experienced during thirty years of Zen training. As you'll see, the integration has hardly begun. There are still wide gaps between what I know of Zen and what I have experienced with patients. But I will be as honest as I can, so that at least I recognize my starting point and can move on from there.

The format I have chosen for this piece of writing is that of a letter, modeled after the letter lying at the heart of the text Fudochi Shimmyo Roku, written by the 17th century Japanese Zen master Takuan to the swordmaster and advisor in strategy to the Shogun of Japan. You have met Takuan before in my story of the Shogun and the tiger.

This text lies at the heart of the training in my lineage of Rinzai Zen Buddhism, articulating some of the most significant concepts from Zen as applied to swordsmanship. I am not Takuan and you are not Yagyu, but I have felt from my supervisory sessions that you easily use the depths of your own experience and spirituality to better understand the ground I stand on. So in some ways, this letter is a continuation of our supervisory conversations.

There are significant concepts from Zen I'd like to explore in describing my personal experience of pastoral care. These are some of the smooth stones in my pocket I keep rubbing as I make my way from patient to patient.

Attachment

Attachment is a fundamental concept of Buddhism. Attachment is seen as that human capacity to ignore the reality of change in order to create some illusion of comfort. We may gain comfort in the short term, but in the end our attachment causes suffering for ourselves and others because change is so damn relentless.

This suffering can be treated superficially by those who would say that all we have to do is let go of our attachments and all will be well. Just live in the flow. Humans have a tremendous capacity to delude themselves, and that is almost ever-present when someone says, "Ah, I have let go."

You heard my "ah-ha!" moment about attachment a week ago when we were reflecting on grief in our small group session. I can't remember which form of grief in myself I was recalling but I was suddenly struck by the way in which the notion of time itself is an attachment.

Chapter XII of the Fudochi text is entitled "Cutting the Before and After" and this phrase is applicable to this concept of attachment to time. In our Zen training, we are continually reminded that time does not flow. There is only now—each moment whole and complete unto itself. That sensation does little good as a belief, but it can become a visceral experience that is cultivated through the practice of Zen calligraphy or a martial art like Kendo. It is, however, extremely hard to live this way. Why? Because we have a strong desire for things to linger.

How many times have I said to a patient, "I'd love to spend more time with you exploring some of these things you just mentioned, but I can't stay longer."? By saying that, I have introduced an artificial concept—that of time—into the conversation. Rather than having the physical sensation that each word might be the last word this patient or I ever utter, there is a desire to know where this story might be going.

This feeling of wanting to know the whole story is natural, but if we think that because it is natural it means time exists, we are deluded. Only if we recognize that we are consciously acting in a deluded fashion do we have a chance of avoiding attachment.

Let's shift to a more profound example of a lack of attachment in a Zen teacher. The teacher in question is the great 18th century Japanese Zen master Hakuin and the story describes an incident when he was the abbot of the temple Shoin-ji.

A young woman who belonged to the temple congregation became pregnant. When her strict father learned of this, he bullied her to name her lover. Thinking that if she blamed a priest she might escape punishment, she told him: "It is Zen master Hakuin." The father said no more, but when the time came and the child was born, he at took the baby to Hakuin, saying, "It seems this is your child." And he piled on insult after insult.

In response, Hakuin only said, "Oh, is that so?" and took the baby into his arms. Thereafter, at all hours and in all weather he would go out to beg milk from the neighboring houses. Wherever Hakuin went, he took the baby, wrapped in the sleeve of his ragged robe. Many of the monks training at Sho-in-ji turned against him and left.

Meanwhile, the mother found she could not bear the agony of separation from her child. And she feared how her lie would be judged in the next world. Finally, she confessed the name of the real father of the child.

Her own father, whose strictness included a strong moral code of right and wrong, became almost mad with fear. He rushed to Hakuin and flattened himself on the ground, begging for for-giveness. The Zen master this time too said only: "Oh, is that so?" and gave him the child.

We already spoke of this story as a great example of non-re-action, an ideal lack of anxiety. But I would do us both a disservice if I left things at that. In reality, this story is not an example of non-reaction in a skilled and psychological-ly mature individual. In ordinary language, Hakuin simply shows no attachment as to whether he is right or wrong in this story. In a Zen perspective, he is viewed as acting out of no-self, a concept that goes beyond that of an "individual."

Self and no-self
This language of self and no-self is difficult. The discus-sion of self and no-self is difficult. But it is critical for understanding Zen Buddhism. I'll start with a memory

about the day my daughter Laura found her ego.

She was three years old, sitting in her high chair in the corner of the dining room. There was the usual mix of food in the mouth, food on the floor, food in her hair, food on the walls—a total experience of squashed peas and sweet potatoes. As I fed her, I watched with my usual mix of pleasure and frustration and wonder.

Then, all of the sudden, I saw what seemed to be a protective shell falling over her. Most likely, this was something I picked up in the expression on her face or a shift in her body. Without thought I said to myself, "Ah, I understand. It is too hard to be simply open to all of experience, it is too painful. We need protection to make life bearable."

And that is what had just happened to her. She found that she could create a form of protection that would make life less raw. All of this—the rapid shift in her way of being and my immediate interpretation of that shift— had happened in an instant.

In the days following this experience, I tried to sort it out. I told myself that this must be natural for all of us. We are not born with an ego, but we find that we need some form of protection as we make sense of the chaos surrounding us.

I also realized that, as we grow up, we forget that, at some point early in our life, we all did what Laura had just done. We create an ego. But creating the ego is not the problem. It seems like a useful thing to have as we learn to make sense of ourselves, other people and the world around us.

But forgetting that we created the ego is the problem. Once we have matured and can better navigate the raw world we live in, we can dismantle that ego. Actually, I should say that we may never dismantle that ego once constructed, but we can see through it and thus not be caught by it.

Another way to talk about self and no-self is to first picture an old-fashioned electric fan, the kind with four metal blades enclosed in a wire cage. Those blades represent the "self." At rest, each blade is solid with a clear delineation of what is blade and what is not-blade. Similarly, I may walk around my everyday life with a clear sense of what is myself and what is not.

But I need to be careful with the fan analogy. While blade and no-blade are clear opposites, self and no-self are not. Once we shift to a Zen perspective, no-self must include self. Otherwise, it remains dualistic.

Another way to say this is that once the fan is turned on, you can no longer see the blades. While both are present, there is no longer a distinction between blade and no-blade. But, if you thought you had now achieved total no-blade by turning on the fan, you would quickly find out how mistaken you were if you tried to reach through the whirling fan to the other side.

Similarly, if you think you have achieved something called no-self, you would be deluded. Self is still present. You can't have one without the other. But when self is unattached to anything, it becomes harder to see.

Let's go back to the ego as I introduced it when I spoke

about my young daughter eating her smashed peas. We often think of ego as a problem, as a barrier to something truer or more fundamental. We might say for example, "Oh, that was just his ego talking," the implication being that behind the ego there is a more fundamental, less self-ish, version of that person.

From a Zen point of view, we would say that you can't separate ego and non-ego. Each creates the other. Fundamentally, it doesn't matter if the ego is still there, but it matters profoundly if you remain attached to it. That would be like trying to only see the fan blades as they start to spin once the fan is turned on. You know that the blades are still there, and you know the space between the blades is still there. But once they are spinning, they are part of each other.

Here is how the late Cistercian monk Thomas Merton explained this difference between the self and no-self when writing about the experience of Christian mystics:

> *The mystical consciousness of St. Theresa implies a certain basic attitude toward the self. The thinking and feeling and willing self is not the starting point of all verifiable reality and of all experience. The primal truth, the ground of all being and truth, is in God the Creator of all that is. The starting point of all Christian belief and experience (in this context) is the primal reality of God as Pure Actuality...*
>
> *The self-centered awareness of the ego is of course a pragmatic psychological reality, but once*

there has been an inner illumination of pure reality, an awareness of the Divine, the empirical self is seen by comparison to be "nothing," that is to say contingent, evanescent, relatively unreal...

To understand this attitude, we have to remember that in this view of things Being is not an abstract objective idea but a fundamental concrete intuition directly apprehended in a personal experience that is incontrovertible and inexpressible. (Zen and the Birds of Appetite, New Directions, 1968. p 26)

That "thinking and feeling and willing self" is what I am calling the self. That "awareness of the Divine" would be the no-self.

Where I disagree with Merton is with his phrase expressing that the empirical self is "relatively unreal." That would be like trying to reach through a moving fan because you think that the fan blades are relatively unreal. Bad idea. Being unattached doesn't mean denying the existence of something. It means seeing through that something.

With these things now said, let's look again at this phrase "no-self." If one is not attached to the self, the self/no-self is free to roam at will, without attachments.

Lao Tzu, whose writings became the foundation of organized Taoism in China, said, "If we learn, we gain in knowledge day by day. If we act according to the Way [Merton's "awareness of the Divine"], we lose day by day. We keep losing until we no longer possess anything to do. In non-action we do everything."

The Tang Dynasty Chinese Zen Master Zhaozhou said the same thing, "I entered Buddhist life when I was a small boy. I have grown old now. Confronted with people, I now find myself powerless to save them. I used to discipline myself in order to help people some day when I became enlightened. Contrary to my expectation, however, I have become a fool whether you believe it or not."

To me, these two statements, one by a Zen master and one by a Taoist, point to the workings of the no-self that goes beyond the psychological concept of non-reaction.

Non-reaction still acts within a concrete individual, someone defined as being the locus of action. There is no question that becoming a non-reactive individual represents a high degree of skill in a mature human being. And, Jeff, that is exactly the kind of hospital chaplains you work so hard to develop.

But that non-reactive chaplain is not the same as the no-self I am struggling to describe. The evidence of the working of the no-self is that there is "nobody in need of saving." While I may not have been aware of it at the time, I think this was a point I was trying make in my story about the mystical hospital, the monk, and the sound of the cello. Do you remember the caravan?

For all of us, patients and travelers alike, with each step we became more transparent, more of the sandstone and the sky showing through us. With each pulse of a step, each pulse of a note, we became more transparent. And our breathing became longer and

*deeper, closer and closer to becoming the wind that
had begun to stir as the first hints of dusk came on.*

*You couldn't tell when it happened, but at a
certain moment, if you had looked away and now
looked back, all of us, camels, horsemen, monks, dogs,
dissolved into sandstone and sky and air. Yet still you
could still hear the cello, and all had been healed.*

Having lived with my Zen teacher for so many years, I
watched him heal duality all day in all that he encountered. And somehow, I could tell that he himself was not
doing anything. There wasn't a healer and someone being healed. There was just healing. That's what Merton,
Lao Tzu, Zhaozhou, and now I have been saying. The self
of the healer is dissolved into something greater.

Shugyo

Having spent so much time talking self and no-self, attachment and no attachment, I need to say something
about the means by which Zen training cultivates a deep
understanding of what is the same and what is different
about those seemingly opposite pairs of words. In other
words, what are the means by which one resolves duality?

In my second theological reflection paper, I wrote
about such means when discussing shugyo, a Japanese
word sometimes translated as "the most rigorous form
of spiritual discipline."

Given that shugyo helps one begin to dissolve duality,
it should make sense that the first duality to be resolved is

that of the mind-body split. This means that, by definition, the work has to be intensely physical. Or a better expression would be to say that you have to throw everything you have into the struggle: your injured right knee, good memories of childhood Christmases, the long breaths and short breaths, everything. Nothing is held back. The point of this intense physicality is to drive the learning into one's bones so that is available at all times under all conditions.

There's an even tougher duality: that of self and other. In a monastic setting, the means of assaulting that is to place the needs of others ahead of your own. That means that all that seems necessary for comfort is challenged: physical comfort, emotional comfort, spiritual comfort. The instruction to "set the needs of others before your own" sounds good, sounds virtuous, but only until you recognize that the unspoken part of the rule is "all the time." The rule must be relentless because the natural human ability to seek comfort is relentless.

The problem with this very human need for comfort comes when those who need comfort seek to ease the suffering of those who are suffering. The point isn't to be uncomfortable. The point is to not be stuck on whether there is comfort or discomfort at any point. We train in order to be free to work from either position without being attached to it.

The experience of undergoing shugyo is difficult. I adapted to the physicality of Zen training—the little sleep and absence of free time—but adapting to the fundamental challenge to my sense of self took longer. Out of my three years in the monastery, it seems as if the second of those years was spent with the unshakable sensation that I was wearing one of those old-fashioned diving helmets. It was if there was a small pane of thick glass between me and the surrounding environment. My senses were narrowed. My ability to communicate intelligibly was limited.

Looking back at that sensation, it showed how limiting my self identity had been up to that point. Without knowing how thoroughly grounded I was in my ego, it was impossible to imagine stepping outside that boundary.

Why would anyone think this degree of spiritual discipline might be a good idea? As my Zen teacher pointed out, it is not uncommon for people late in their lives to resolve this boundary between self and other. They easily seem to set the needs of others ahead of their own. The problem, however, is that this phase of their life before dying is relatively short. So one goal of undergoing shugyo is to accelerate the learning process so that before we die we have more time to take care of people, to address human suffering.

Suffering and Zen

Suffering lies at the heart of Buddhism, by tradition being the first teaching the Buddha offered following his enlightenment. The story told is that Buddha sought out the five ascetics that he had trained with during his years of extreme austerity, teaching them what are called the Four Noble Truths.

In my own lineage of Zen, we would teach what

the Buddha discerned about the nature of suffering but would not declare them "truths." That word implies something to believe. For a Zen person, these things only have meaning once experienced, and experienced in your bones. We might say:

- To be alive is to experience suffering. (The first "truth")
- The experience of suffering occurs because we are attached. Attached to ideas, to things, to illusions and delusions, to people, to a sense of who and what we are. (The second "truth")
- To become detached from any of those does not lead to an end of suffering. Rather it is transcending the duality of attachment/ detachment that leads to an end of suffering. And the end of suffering still can include grief and sorrow as well as peace and joy. (The third "truth")
- The method of transcending duality is through shugyo, severe mind-body training. (The fourth "truth")

What is Zen?

Though this may seem a backwards way of writing, I feel that we now can better pick up this question of "What is Zen?" Tanouye Roshi describes Zen as a verb, not a noun. It is not a religion but the act of training in breath and posture such that placing the needs of others ahead of your own, continually, seems the most natural thing in the world.

Other Zen teachers' descriptions of Zen seem less useful so I won't go into that literature. But I do like the ways in which Thomas Merton wrestled with this same question, speaking as a highly empathic outsider to the world of Zen.

The whole aim of Zen is not to make foolproof statements about experience, but to come to direct grips with reality without the mediation of logical verbalizing. But what reality? There is certainly a kind of living and non-verbal dialectic in Zen between the ordinary everyday experience of the senses (which is by no means arbitrarily repudiated) and the experience of enlightenment.

Zen is not an idealistic rejection of sense and matter in order to ascend to a supposedly invisible reality which alone is real. The Zen experience is a direct grasp of the unity of the invisible and the visible. (Zen and the Birds of Appetite, New Directions, 1968. p 37)

Everything I've written so far, and anything I would write about these topics all point to the same thing: the nature of a non-dualistic reality.

This reality is impossible to write about—it can only be shown or lived. That showing can be poems, ink on paper, the sound of chanting, the feeling from a dish of fresh vegetables, the way in which you take your bath. But still, that is all too easy to say and of little use to others. And I am sidestepping an important question: Have I been a Hakuin to any patient in this hospital? Not Hakuin the non-reactive self, but Hakuin the no-self.

I would love to play out some wondrous examples from these past three months, but I don't have any. Instead. I just have glimpses of this, the times when I was unconscious of there being anything particular to do and yet much seemed to happen.

You said something important yesterday during supervision. You said, "I have stepped through the looking glass and, once I did that, there is no turning back." I woke up last night to those words, thinking how inadequate this letter feels in showing my experience of stepping through the looking glass.

The feeling your statement evoked for me is similar to that which occurs within me when the koans—the paradoxes of my Zen tradition—are resolved. That is an experience of stepping through a looking glass. And one that permanently rearranges one's bone structure.

But this notion of "there is no turning back...." Why has it been easier for me during CPE to feel that I am training my self, training my cognitive abilities, my emotional abilities, my empathic abilities? Easier than training my no-self? Whatever happened in "finishing" my koan training (the quotation marks are there because we never actually finish our work with koan), I'm still stepping back and forth through that looking glass as I work with patients.

I don't have an adequate answer. But at least now I have better language for wrapping up. In this letter, I have avoided what perhaps was expected, a summary of my learning with patients.

Instead, I have been exploring the gap between the high

standard of healing I know from my Zen tradition and the kind of healing I am capable of providing. Your colleague at my initial interview seemed worried that I was being too hard on myself with my expression of the standards I wanted to hold myself to. There, I said that the work of a Zen priest was to take away fear. To take away fear means to take away the need for a dualistic framework of reality—a need, for example, of life and death as opposites, for self and other to be opposites. And to do that work, it means that I can't be caught in that same dualistic framework.

That is a wonderfully difficult standard. It has no value in the abstract, only in the moment by moment. Perhaps what is different now, as compared to that day talking with my interviewers, is that I have my answer to your recent question. When I finished presenting my report about the two brothers—"seeing the pebbles on the bottom"—and you asked, "So what is available to you now?" I answered "...stupidity...ignorance" with some sense of wonder.

The wonder is that I should admit such things to myself, a product of so many years of great education. But looking at that exchange now, I can better see that I can at least glimpse the experience "in non-action, we do everything" that Lao Tzu expressed and that Tanouye Roshi exemplified.

That's all for now - Gordon

12.
Please take care of me.

I t all seems so neat – this narrative arc of my three months of chaplaincy training. The time started with my excitement about learning intensely, and with my emotional armor well in place. Five weeks later, I hit crisis, doubt and despair as my armor shredded. And then a sense of innocence and wonder as I came out the other side feeling naked. As you read in the last chapter, I also began to consolidate and articulate a clearer sense of what it means to be a Zen chaplain.

But I use that phrase "so neat" cautiously. Even though I began my chaplain training with a high degree of motivation and many years of life experience and health care experience behind me, three months was really only enough to help me find what a beginner in this work of facing suffering I am.

Ian was a young man admitted to the hospital for alcohol detoxification. I met with him twice in one day—morning and afternoon—in his hospital room, with no visitors present. I expected there to be at least one more visit with Ian the following morning after I came back on service. But instead, during our morning briefing, I found him on the discharge list. He had left against medical advice in the early morning, with his nurse writing in his chart, with considerable emotion between the lines, about her concerns for this patient.

If there even is such a thing, Ian was no ordinary alcoholic/drug user. Certainly, his story was more extreme than most. At fifteen, he had—in vain—tried to resuscitate his mother after a drug overdose. Since her death, Ian had watched or participated in three more resuscitation efforts on people close to him.

The two most recent had happened just this year. In April, he awoke to find his pregnant fiancée Andrea on her hands and knees, seemingly choking to death. The ambulance and the emergency crew arrived 27 minutes later, but she was already dead. Two weeks later, he found his older brother Phil unconscious on the floor, turning blue. Phil had been upset that his girlfriend had left him. Like their mother, Ian's brother overdosed. Unlike their mother, Phil survived.

Ian had been an alcoholic and a drug user before his fiancée Andrea died but his use since was harder and now included heroin. He told me that if, by committing suicide, he could be with Andrea in any meaningful way, he would take his life as easily as flipping a light switch.

Ian's hospital chart notes showed he was there for treatment for an acute detoxification incident following heavy alcohol use. But to me, this was clearly a patient who also needed treatment for extreme despair.

The primary work of the two visits with Ian had been to help him find his strength, to help him be open to his love of his fiancée, no longer living and by his side.

Verbally, I had told Ian that he was a strong man if he could still be standing after the many tragedies in his life. And verbally I told him to make a place in his heart for his dead fiancée, so she could keep returning there to feel his love and receive comfort. (Ian had recounted a visit from Andrea's spirit a few months earlier and longed for her to return in the same fashion.)

I had been speaking words to Ian about these things but in a deeper fashion I was doing all that I could physically to reinforce his strength. I watched some of that emerge over the course of our two conversations, seeing his face take on strength, seeing his body look less defeated.

It was similar with the discussion of making a place in his heart for his dead fiancée. Non-verbally I had to show him what this feeling is like, showing him how I have done this in my own body for people I have loved and lost.

Perhaps because these visits with the patient were so physical, I was primed to do the same with his discharge nurse. Going up to the unit the morning after, it had been an easy question to ask, "When will Fran (Ian's nurse of the night before) be coming back on service? I'd like to check in with her about the patient who left AMA last night and see how she is doing." When the nurse on service answered, her relaxed body language showed that she was touched that I would want to know how one of her colleagues was doing. I felt that this nurse was encouraging me, "Please take care of Fran." And she gave me Fran's home phone number.

My first impulse was, "I can't call her. She is off-service." But the nurse I was talking to encouraged me, telling me that Fran had young children and that she spent time with them in the morning before she herself got some sleep. I called her.

Fran seemed surprised at first that I had called, but she quickly got into the conversation. She described her fears for this patient's well-being, her frustration when he left against medical advice, and her sadness at the many losses in his life.

She spoke of the confusion she had felt when Ian's younger brother Phil phoned before Ian left the hospital. He said, "Please don't let him go," meaning Ian. Fran told me that Phil sounded intoxicated on the phone, so she didn't know if she should believe all that he was telling her. Later, she got a call from the Emergency Room: a Madison police officer had found Ian "looking lost," wandering the streets at 4:30 am while still wearing his Meriter Hospital bracelet.

Fran sounded proud that she had done all she could on Ian's behalf before he left against medical advice, or maybe it was pride that she could still care about him after he left the hospital. She welcomed the chance to talk about him with me, knowing I shared her worries for the patient.

I felt something akin to a sense of wonder. I had gone to the patient's unit of the hospital with a vague need to talk with Ian's last nurse and to offer comfort, but I had not anticipated this moving phone conversation. Still, given a form of permission from the nurse I did talk with at the hospital, it felt easy and natural to call Fran, explaining who I was and why I was calling.

This was the first time I felt that I had effectively provided care to a nurse. And Fran's need for care wasn't simply handed to me. I had to care enough about Ian to search for his discharge notes. I had to read the emotions between the lines of the discharge note Fran wrote in order to realize that she might need care. I had to look for her, ask for help finding her, and then actually call her. All these steps seem like perfectly natural ones to take, but they hadn't come naturally to me.

I watched a startled reaction from Jeff when recounting these events during the next day's supervisory session. When I told him that I called Fran at home, I could see him doing a rapid mental scan to evaluate whether or not this act was appropriate.

His startled reaction helped me in turn to ask myself if at any point making this phone call seemed inappropriate. The answer for myself was "no," but that was surprising because I had never followed up on a patient in this way. Yet it had all seemed so natural.

The primary permission must have come from the day nurse's body language as she encouraged me to call Fran. That feeling of "Please take care of her" was also a feeling of "Should the time come, please take care of me." And I can recognize within myself and my actions a similar feeling of "Should the time come, please take care of me." There was a primal recognition that we all seek someone to take care of us, someone to take us in their arms and say, "It's OK. I'm here now. I won't leave you. You are going to be OK."

Writing now, I'm surprised to find myself in tears, but here they are. I've tapped into something deep between myself and Ian and these nurses. I'm finding something that we all share: the need to be able to say, "Please take care of me." And to then have someone respond.

Looking back at Ian and his nurse Fran, these lessons don't seem spiritual or pastoral or theological. They seem human. I could get all Buddhist now and begin exploring the words "Please take care of me," examining the way in which just by asking such a thing, some form of healing becomes available because it shows that desire to ease the gap between self and other. Just by expressing that desire, the gap begins to narrow.

But at the moment, that Buddhist explication seems out of place. Instead, I'm thinking back to that Bodhisatva of Compassion and the translation of its Sanskrit

name: The Regarder of the Cries of the World. That regarding, that listening, doesn't feel theological. It's hard
physical work. It's manual labor. And when done right,
it feels human.

13.
I am not an animal!

Lacy was a freckle-faced 39-year-old woman with short red/blond hair, lying on the gurney in Room 4 of the Emergency Room. When I first met her, she wore dark-rimmed glasses, had a cast on her left forearm and a walking splint on her right leg. Her parents had driven her to the hospital because she had suddenly lost vision in her left eye. They feared she might have experienced a stroke.

Medical staff response to a potential stroke is skilled and rapid, with lots of information gathered and evaluated so any necessary treatment can begin as quickly as possible. But in the midst of the questions, the numbers, the medications, the equipment, there was an anguished cry, "I am not an animal!"

For a moment, all was still.

It was Lacy's voice. With no vision in her left eye, she could not see the nurse standing on that side of the bed, asking her questions. Lacy heard only a disembodied voice. She was confused by all the elements of the neurologist's examination. After being touched various ways and asked to describe what she felt, she asked the doctor, "What do you want me to feel?" Lacy was overwhelmed, unable to control the chaotic scene. But at least she knew that she was human.

Unlike most people, she had a great deal of experience with emergency rooms and hospitals. This was her fifteenth visit to this hospital in the past eleven months. She had been admitted to the hospital five times in the past eleven months. At age nine, Lacy had been diagnosed with a rare form of diabetes, sometimes called "brittle" diabetes because of the high degree of difficulty in managing blood sugar levels.

But manage those sugars Lacy had for the past three decades. When a decision was made in the ER to start giving her insulin following standard protocols, she got upset all over again. She tried to describe to the medical staff what had happened to her glucose levels in the past when deviating from her own insulin regimen. It turned out that she was not having a stroke, so everyone began listening to her in ways that had seemed difficult before. And the sense of emergency lessened.

My impression as I watched this occur was that Lacy needed a sense of control, and she needed respect. Admiring her strength in articulating her needs in a hospital setting, I was ready to provide that respect. Lacy was firm and clear.

Given a final assignment to complete before finishing my three months of hospital training, I asked Lacy for permission to focus that report on her medical needs, her psychological needs, and her spiritual needs as she lived with this difficult-to-manage disease.

When I saw her the next day following admission, she was much more relaxed and apologized for any harshness I might have felt from her answers to my questions in the emergency room. With an odd, somewhat hoarse voice, she spoke easily and readily about her history of diabetes and the ways in which she has learned to manage her life. Despite her age, she had a childlike quality, perhaps from the sense of innocence when she spoke of things she liked, and also by her tendency to rapidly cycle between anger and happiness. She seemed to make rapid judgments about those people she could trust and those she could not.

She agreed to participate in my case review study, and we met several times over the next few days: sometimes just the two of us, and sometimes with her parents.

All people with diabetes experience swings in their blood sugar levels, primarily because they don't produce the regulating hormone called insulin in a normal fashion. As compared to people without diabetes, most patients with insulin-dependent diabetes have roughly 50 percent the amount of insulin to help control their blood sugars. What made Lacy's condition harder to manage was that her baseline was closer to only ten percent of the normal amount of insulin—meaning that any changes in blood sugar were all the more dramatic.

According to her parents, Lacy has had "hundreds" of hospitalizations since her initial diagnosis. That may be an exaggeration, but I could find records for 55 admissions to our hospital over the past ten years and numerous additional visits to the Emergency Room with problems that did not require admission. Lacy said the biggest impact of having this form of diabetes is that "my body is different every day, just like the weather."

For example, in her physician's admitting note, he listed the following conditions in her past medical history:

> *Pancreatitis, Diabetes Melitus type 1, Chronic kidney disease, Unspecified asthma, Hypothyroidism, Breakdown of skin tissue, Neuropathy – extremities and in GI tract, history of MRSA, Cellulitis, Dermatopsychosis, Diabetic gastroparesis, Celiac disease–possible, Diabetic ketoacidosis–recurrent, Dyslipedemia, Hypertension, Primary ovarian failure, Major depression, Generalized anxiety disorder, Osteoporosis, Migraine headache, Non-alcoholic steatohepatitis.*

That's a lot of weather. Her father had run a dairy farm for 35 years but said he now had an easier life since he began raising beef cattle. He also said, "I once was rich one way [selling milk], and now I'm rich another way [in his relationship with his daughter]." The implication was that Lacy's medical expenses over the years have been very high.

Both parents describe, with a bit of wonder in their voices, how they got through the early years, trying to find physicians who could understand their ailing daughter's glucose fluctuations. They described firing one early medical team out of frustration. There was also a low point when they thought Lacy would die. They had also been told she would most likely only live until age 28 or 29.

Talking further about Lacy's own understanding of her condition, her father said that Lacy asked him several years ago to talk to a funeral home director so that they could figure out her funeral arrangements. And he did. Both parents felt that she was much more ready to die than they were ready to have her die.

Her education has been disrupted continually since age nine. Lacy said that she didn't have many friends but was close to her family and those in an elementary school where she does voluntary work.

As for her spiritual tradition, she was raised a Lutheran and still considered that her faith. She had a fairly pragmatic view of her faith, as best exemplified by a question she asked her aunt when this aunt reported that she had seen an angel standing by her bed the previous evening. Our young woman's response to her aunt had been a matter-of-fact, "What kind?"

Given all this, what did I actually do for Lacy? The term "brittle diabetes" is controversial. Some physicians see it more as a behavioral or psychological difficulty in managing insulin than an inherently medical problem. If that first perspective can be validated, then what is the role of spiritual care in resolving that behavioral difficulty? But if the condition is organic, a scientifically-verified variation of the more common forms of diabetes, then spiritual care could be more a matter of coping with chronic problems, rather than resolving the condition itself.

I was too much of a beginner to choose one approach over the other. I started as an explorer, wondering how I might help her and in the process what I might learn about spiritual care.

Pastoral care for a patient can be something like a jazz improvisation; based on some sort of theme, a great deal of exploration goes on. It can be hard to discern the structure of that improvisation while it is happening. Similarly, the work of a chaplain with a patient and family can seem to be occurring without much structure.

However, three interwoven phases of care become more obvious in retrospect. These phases are: developing an empathic relationship with the patient, assessing the patient's spiritual needs (making a spiritual "diagnosis"), then working to best meet those needs. Given the nature of this work, all three phases can take time, and sufficient time is often not readily available. That was the case with Lacy, but let's look examine these phases of care, nevertheless.

Phase 1: the essence of this phase is active listening as the patient describes their life, their problems, their dreams. By "active," I mean a whole body form of attention that is meant to attend to the verbal content of a discussion, the verbal structure and format (word choice, pauses, sequence of topics), as well as all non-verbal forms of communication.

Through this form of listening, a sensitive form of exploration takes place, working to answer the question, "What is important to this patient?" In Lacy's case, the overwhelming answer that emerged from my conversations with her was control and respect. This is what I heard in her cry, "I am not an animal!" and all subsequent conversations reinforced that impression.

Phase 2: In this phase, the work is to examine how needs for control and respect fit into a framework that could be addressed through spiritual care; in other words, what a chaplain contributes to her care. One framework for this perspective comes from a study of patients in crisis. Patient experiences revealed a set of categories that seemed to encompass the various kinds of spiritual or existential dilemma that patients may find themselves in. Examples include religious apathy, religious denial, and religious vengeance. Also, religious doubt, anger at God, conflict with church dogma.

For Lacy and her parents, at first glance there were no noticeable spiritual dilemmas. The degree of faith they had seemed adequate for dealing with the problems that they faced with her brittle diabetes. Each of them had come into some form of equilibrium.

But here's where things get difficult: Lacy's equilibrium did not seem to be a particularly powerful one, one that was grounded after a deep exploration of the meaning of her life. She had, and her parents as well, accepted that she was going to die from the impact of diabetes on one of her organ systems, sooner rather than later.

We could perhaps say "All is as well as it could be. What more is there to do?" As a chaplain, however, I'm not content leaving things at that. I say this for two reasons: one spiritual, one practical.

On the practical side, I was concerned that Lacy's medical needs and hospitalizations will become more and more frequent. None of us know when she will be able to say, "There is nothing more to do. I'm ready to die." Without clarity about this, Lacy may be swept deeper into an arena in which she loses more and more control, and perhaps more and more respect—these things she needs the most.

Another practical concern is the role stress may play in her glucose control crises—an issue emphasized by those who treat patients with this suite of symptoms. We don't have to be conscious of stress for it to have a major impact on the function of all bodily systems. Stress can be just as powerful when we are unaware of it. So, if I could find out what stresses Lacy might be experiencing, I might be able to help her better address those, and perhaps lessen the impact of stress on glucose levels.

On the spiritual side, with more time I would want to know what Lacy's experience of transcendence has been. Has she ever felt the presence of the Divine? Has she looked deeply at the meaning of her life, especially in the context of her family? Is she at peace with the ways in which her medical condition has taken over her life since age nine?

Human beings have a phenomenal capacity to cope, to accommodate, to tell ourselves stories that make things seem all right. But that is not always the healthiest condition for our spirit to be in.

Phase 3: As a chaplain, I would summarize my concern for Lacy by saying, "She is coping with her illness; she is not yet healed of her illness." Obviously, I don't mean "healed" medically, but that it is possible for her to feel whole and complete as a human being despite all the damage to her body. So, given more time with her, how would I proceed?

Let's look at the dark side of "control." There lies vulnerability and weakness. I felt neither of these in her on the surface, but I can imagine they may be there. Here's where the therapeutic self of the chaplain becomes most significant. To explain this phrase, "therapeutic self," I'll contrast two approaches to a possible conversation.

In one approach, the focus is all on Lacy. There might be a sensitive exploration of the ways in which she finds her sense of weakness and vulnerability. This is difficult terrain for anyone. And I can imagine that if I simply stood outside this terrain and said, "Why don't you go in and take a look at these uncomfortable things?", then nothing will happen.

In the second approach, the focus would be on the two of us together. "Lacy, I am a confident person in my life. There is not much that scares me anymore. This seems to be true for you as well. But what I know of myself, what I can feel in myself, is that underneath that confidence are my fears.

"Fear of losing control. Fear of losing respect. Fear of being weak. Fear of appearing weak. Fear of hurting others with weakness. Those are as much a part of me as my confidence. They are also what make me whole. It is natural for me or anyone to have those fears. So, Lacy, would you be willing to take a look with me at some of these possible vulnerabilities within you, some of these possible weaknesses?"

I could say those words aloud, depending on the situation. But here is the deep power of the "therapeutic self" mentioned above. If I am deeply aware of my vulnerabilities and weaknesses, then even if I don't mention them or describe them aloud, Lacy will know at a deep level that I have them. This is pure animal instinct that I think all humans have. And by Lacy knowing that I know, she gains courage to face her own fears. She would no longer be alone with her vulnerabilities and fears. After we face those things in Lacy, there would be a chance for her healing.

14.
How does the music
do that?

Presenting Lacy's case to my chaplain colleagues and hospital staff was the last formal act of three months of CPE. It had been three months of working to develop what I found myself calling a "muscular" form of chaplaincy. A visceral, sensory, physical, manual labor form of chaplaincy.

Before finishing this story of my hospital training, I want to describe why I find that muscular form of chaplaincy so compelling.

I'll start with an address delivered to the parents of the incoming students at the Boston Conservatory by Karl Paulnack, pianist and director of performing arts school's music division. He started his 2004 address by talking in general about the power and value of music, but then got very specific. "The most important concert of my entire life took place in a nursing home in Fargo, North Dakota, about four years ago." Continuing, he said:

I was playing with a very dear friend of mine who is a violinist. We began, as we often do, with Aaron Copland's Sonata [for Violin and Piano], which was written during World War II and dedicated to a young friend of Copland's, a young pilot who was shot down during the war.

Now, we often talk to our audiences about the pieces we are going to play rather than providing them with written program notes. But in this case, because we began the concert with this piece, we decided to talk about the piece later in the program and to just come out and play the music without explanation.

Midway through the piece, an elderly man seated in a wheelchair near the front of the concert hall began to weep. This man, whom I later met, was clearly a soldier. Even in his 70's, it was clear from his buzz-cut hair, square jaw and general demeanor that he had spent a good deal of his life in the military.

I thought it a little bit odd that someone would be moved to tears by that particular movement of that particular piece, but it wasn't the first time I've heard crying in a concert, and we went on with the concert and finished the piece.

When we came out to play the next piece on the program, we decided to talk about both the first and second pieces, and we described the circumstances

*in which the Copland piece was written and men-
tioned its dedication to a downed pilot. With this,
the man in the front of the audience became so disturbed that he had to leave the auditorium.*

*I honestly figured that we would not see him
again, but he did come backstage afterwards, tears
and all, to explain himself. What he told us was this:
"During World War II, I was a pilot, and I was in
an aerial combat situation where one of my team's
planes was hit. I watched my friend bail out, and
watched his parachute open, but the Japanese planes
which had engaged us returned and machine gunned
across the parachute chords so as to separate the
parachute from the pilot, and I watched my friend
drop away into the ocean, realizing that he was lost.*

*I have not thought about this for many years,
but during that first piece of music you played, this
memory returned to me so vividly that it was as
though I was reliving it. I didn't understand why
this was happening, why now, but then when you
came out to explain that this piece of music was
written to commemorate a lost pilot, it was a little
more than I could handle.*

*How does the music do that? How did it find
those feelings and those memories in me?"*

The old pilot's question haunts me: "How does the music
do that?" It haunted my work as a chaplain and my work
as a Zen priest and teacher. Or, to shift to a general form

of that question, "How do we take away suffering?" That is the question I want to explore before ending.

To look at "how" first, we must ask what that particular piece of Copland's music did. It captured something so deeply that it touched a suffering experienced decades earlier. It did that without words, without explanation, without an evocative title such as "Sonata for a Downed Pilot." Something was embodied in the music. But for it to become so well embodied that it worked as it did, it would also have to come out of a certain form of embodiment in Aaron Copland and in the musicians who performed that piece.

I can't speak about this as a composer or a musician, and I can't speak from the perspective of a neuroscientist, but I can speak as someone who has lived a life in the world of Zen. I have seen similar experiences play out in several different ways.

If what I know and what Copland and those musicians accomplished are similar, then I can suggest what that "certain form of embodiment" might be. First, the sorrow that Copland experienced long ago when he lost his pilot friend had to be deep and strong, overwhelming. He would have become a different person after this experience. Something shifted in his breath, his bones.

Then, Copland needed to be a master craftsman; the techniques with which he composed this musical piece had to be of the highest order. For a master craftsman, this means that little ego goes into the work being created. There would be as direct a transmission of emotion into form as is humanly possible. No thoughts of himself, not even thoughts of his friend. Just sorrow.

The test for this level of craftsmanship would be for an astute listener to ask themselves, "When I hear this music, am I hearing Copland as a man, or am I hearing something transcendent?" In other words, "Has Copland disappeared?"

Language is so difficult here. These things need a poet to find the right words to express something with no grounding in words. But, as imperfectly as I've expressed myself, this is something of the "how" this elderly pilot in the audience was so moved.

Likewise, we would have to add something similar about the craftsmanship of the musicians performing the piece. How well could they get out of their own way, just as Copland had to get out of his own way, for them to bring the deep sorrow of so many years ago into a room where that elderly man sat weeping?

The elderly pilot asked, "How does the music do that?" My version was "How do we take away suffering?" To go from his question to my version means that we have to take a logical leap. We have to answer the question, "Did Copland take away suffering from this man by helping him relive his experience?" Everything in me says, "Yes!"

Broad and deep literature has been written on this same question, by psychologists, psychiatrists, and all those professionals who work to heal the many forms of trauma that people can experience. But when I answer "yes" to the above question, I stand only on my experiences during these three months of CPE.

When I face suffering, I ease the suffering of those I face. The act of facing someone in anguish, in and of itself, begins to ease that suffering. We can look at this act in two ways: first in the way I do that facing and secondly in the ways that something is happening in both of us as that facing takes place. Again, words are difficult here, but I want to examine both of those ways.

When I face suffering, it is a highly physical act, as described several times in this book. It involves an intense search within me for a precise form of breath and posture. When I find that form, a deep sense of gravity runs throughout my whole body. It feels like I have optimized something. It's a search informed by decades of training Zen, then tested in my encounters with every variety of patient.

That optimization could be of my hearing. What can I do to tune my sense of hearing most accurately to this person in front of me? That tuning is a physical sensation: How about this?...no, not quite... let me shift my weight this way to get a longer exhalation...getting closer ... and then, Bam! That's it. My sense of self disappears and what's left is sadness and suffering.

But that optimization could also be of my strength, something described when working with Cathy, the mother of Gillian, kept alive in the ICU following her heroin overdose. What physical work do I need to do in order to deliver the most strength possible to another, someone feeling crushed by pain, or doubt, or sorrow? Again, a rapid search goes on as I work physically to get a sensation that, for that moment at least, gives them everything I can possibly give.

So far I am talking as if we've got two people in these scenarios. I am acting in some fashion. I am "facing suffering." Whomever I am facing may not be. They may be simply suffering. But let's examine the act of facing suffering/easing suffering another way.

Start with a person suffering. There are so many forms of suffering but the one that feels most fundamental to me is the sensation of feeling alone. I am alone in this pain. I am alone in this despair. I am alone in this confusion. I am alone in this fear.

When we feel these things we may also be expressing, unconsciously or not, as I did in that encounter with Fran, the nurse who took care of Ian, "Please take care of me."

There are medications that ease pain, prayers that ease despair, words that ease confusion, embraces that take away fear. All of them are answers to "Please take care of me." But I contend that what underlies all of these is a sensation something akin to "I need you to become me."

It sounds so strange, I know, but reflect on this. Think of a time when your mother or your father didn't just understand the pain you were going through but seemed even closer than that. There was a sensation that somehow the pain of the hurt knee or the broken heart was shared; it was no longer just yours. And in that sharing, the suffering shifted. It wasn't so bad. It wasn't going to last forever. Life as you knew it wasn't over. You were not alone.

This was a long route to get back to my statement: "When I face suffering, I ease the suffering of those I face." The physicality of facing suffering gets to the heart of the experience of suffering—namely that experience of feeling alone. I can't explain why, but time and time again the sensation of optimizing my act of facing suffering has let me go inside that experience.

Yes, I have decades of training in that physicality and yes, when faced with testing that ability with hospital patients for three months, I know how much of a beginner I am. I don't speak with pride about such things. But I do speak with a sense of possibility. The suffering in a hospital is a suffering of aloneness and it is possible to heal that aloneness.

The aloneness of Mr. Peterson, the aged insurance salesman, more concerned about the health of his home of 53 years than of his own health. The aloneness of Cathy after Gillian died from a heroin overdose. The aloneness of Ian who watched his pregnant fiancée die when she wasn't resuscitated in time. The aloneness of Grace, that veteran ICU nurse who dealt with so many deaths from heroin overdoses. The aloneness of Lee, recently released from prison, freshly-diagnosed with liver cancer, looking for respect for his skill in surviving a rough life.

We need not stop there. We could speak of the incredible aloneness that physicians experience, given their esoteric knowledge and long years of training. Who can possibly understand their experience other than another physician? Or how about the aloneness of the director of a spiritual care program in a hospital, as he struggles to prove the value that spiritual care provides to patients, quantifying value with dollars and cents something that defies such quantification? Or the aloneness of a hospital administrator trying to figure out how to pay for the care of people with no insurance.

I've wandered far afield here from my chaplain training experience, but once you start viewing human behavior through a lens called "being alone," it is hard to stop.

I also want to describe an entirely different answer to the question, "How do we take away suffering?" After perhaps giving you as much Zen Buddhism as you can stand, let's hear a useful Christian answer.

This comes from the current Archbishop of Canterbury, Justin Welby, in a speech given to the Council on Foreign Relations in Washington, D.C. He spoke on many subjects, including the difficult work that the Anglican Church does in Africa as it works to bring about reconciliation in the face of widespread religious violence.

At the end of his talk, Welby was asked what skills someone needed in order to face the amount and degree of suffering created by such religious conflicts. How can someone possibly remain effective in the face of so much suffering? His answer was stunning:

You have to let your heart be broken. You've got to let your heart be broken by encountering people where they are...Part of the dialogue that we need is a dialogue that involves great pain. We must let ourselves be hurt.

What I find remarkable in this statement is the expression of a unity between the person suffering and the person facing that suffering. Welby says people facing pain must let themselves be hurt. However, that is not just something that happens to someone: that they hurt when they encounter someone who is hurting. The "training," if you will, for a person entering that encounter, is to voluntarily let their heart be broken.

We might survive the experience of a broken heart. We might sympathize with someone with a broken heart. But who might think that would be a good idea, "to let their heart be broken?" Who in their right mind would voluntarily let their heart be broken?

The Archbishop of Canterbury, with heartfelt and painful experience behind him, would say this is a good idea. As would I. Most likely Aaron Copland didn't ask for his heart to be broken by a friend dying. But broken it was, and because of that he created something that showed he faced suffering in a deeply physical way. And because Copland faced it, decades later he was able to ease the suffering of a man in the front row of performance of Copland's creation.

A chaplaincy of embodiment; that's what I learned is possible. We've explored different ways that suffering can be embodied, then faced. It might take the form it took in Copland, though he would never have wished for it to happen. Or it might take the form suggested by Justin Welby, to let ourselves be hurt so we can face suffering.

This Zen guy would say the work of facing suffering is manual labor—hard work that can make you sweat. A chaplain can become a therapeutic instrument, bringing training into a patient's room within your bones. If your bones are in the room, then all that you have learned and experienced is available to your patient.

This is what happened when Mrs. Baker, the elderly woman lying in the darkness, answered my question, "How are you doing?" by saying, "I have lost so much in my life." If you remember, less than two hours before this encounter, I myself finally truly felt how much I had lost in my life.

When facing suffering, let yourself disappear. It is one of the great paradoxes that the more fully you know yourself–your strengths, your fears, your vulnerabilities–the less need there is for that "you" to be present. Copeland was a master craftsman whose ego lost its grip. And when we encounter the products of such craftsmanship, we instinctively feel there is little attachment to ego.

With a sense of wonder at my own words – words that didn't actually feel like they were mine as I wrote them at the start of my training – I come at last to my conclusion as to what chaplaincy can be:

Healing happens but there is no healer present.

Now, remembering a story from the early days of chaplaincy training...

...For all of us, patients and travelers alike, with each step we became more transparent, more of the sandstone and the sky showing through us. With each pulse of a step, each pulse of a note, we became more transparent. And our breathing became longer and deeper, closer and closer to becoming the wind that had begun to stir as the first hints of dusk came on.

You couldn't tell when it happened, but at a certain moment, if you had looked away and now looked back, all of us, camels, horsemen, monks, dogs, dissolved into sandstone and sky and air. Yet still you could still hear the cello, and all had been healed.

Acknowledgements

This book focuses on only three months of my life as a hospital chaplain, but those months felt so compelling to write about because they gave me such a highly condensed experience of many decades of my life. That makes the acknowledgement process meaningful but difficult.

Each of those decades had me learning from great teachers and colleagues but also had me learning as I taught countless students and served countless patients. All names of the patients included in my stories here have been altered to protect their identity.

In the world of chaplaincy, Jeff Billerbeck was a very important influence. And the fuel I brought to chaplaincy came out of my Zen training, work that began when I met Tenshin Tanouye Roshi in 1978. I could begin bringing this training out into the world when I was hired in 1993 into the newly-formed Department of Family Medicine at the University of Hawaii by Curtis Takemoto-Gentile. This medical school setting is where my public focus on how we learn to suffer first emerged.

I'm grateful for the opportunities I had to explore that focus through short-term teaching opportunities at Williams College, Oxford University, the University of San Francisco, and the University of Wisconsin in addition to the fifteen years I taught at the University of Hawaii.

Other significant colleagues from these intersecting worlds include Seiji Yamada, Jayson Estby, and John Frey, each of whom read an earlier draft of this manuscript. Kay Bauman, Lu Marchand and Jen Nehls provided highly empathic role models as I was learning both to teach and to heal.

My training partners in chaplaincy were Craig Simenson, Lisa Schoenwetter, Stuart McCoy and Margit Sande-Kerback as well as fellow Night Chaplains at Meriter Hospital. Paula McKenzie was a gentle guide for professional work as a hospital chaplain in a Catholic hospital. Kenneth Kushner, family medicine faculty member and fellow Zen teacher, wrote the letter of recommendation that brought me into the world of Family Medicine and has nurtured my work ever since.

The writing of this book began during a workshop offered by Laurie Scheer, a constant source of encouragement for telling my story. Veronica Rueckert helped me capture more of that story through heartfelt interviews that resulted in a video series on facing suffering. Dana Isaacson was a thorough editor to this book and Zachary Opaskar gave shape and format to my words through his book design.

As you will read, my children Laura, Alex and Sam gave me the motivation to learn all that I can about facing suffering. And my wife Patricia was that essential voice for any writer, a never-failing "Please write this book."

Behind those whom I have named, I see the faces of countless others and I am grateful to all.

About the author

Gordon Greene is the Head Priest at the Spring Green Zen Dojo in southwestern Wisconsin. He is also Clinical Professor of Family Medicine at the University of Wisconsin School of Medicine and Public Health. His author website (gordongreene.org) includes a number of essays, videos, and links on the topic of facing suffering. He can be reached at gmgreene@wisconsinzen.org.

Lightning Source UK Ltd.
Milton Keynes UK
UKHW040748281022
411251UK00004B/312